CARE

For One Another

CARE

For One Another

Biblical Caregiving Principles

CHARLES PUCHTA

Published by:

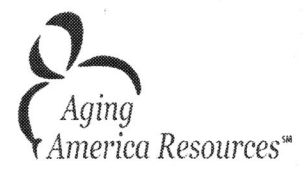

Aging America Resources℠

Cincinnati

Copyright © 2005-2009 Charles Puchta, Aging America Resources, Inc.

Cover design by John Acree, Redeemed Design

2009 Edition, 3rd Printing

All rights reserved. No part of this publication may be reproduced, stored in a retrieval system, or transmitted in any form or by any means, digital, electronic, mechanical, photocopying, recording, or otherwise, or conveyed via the Internet or a website without prior written permission from Aging America Resources, Inc.

Inquires should be addressed to
Aging America Resources
11611 Kosine Lane, Suite 105
Loveland, OH 45140-1912

ISBN: 978-0-9722104-8-5

Printed in the United States of America

Library of Congress Control Number: Pending

All scripture quotations, unless otherwise indicated, are taken from the HOLY BIBLE, NEW INTERNATIONAL VERSION®. NIV®. Copyright ©1973, 1978, 1984 by International Bible Society. Used by permission of Zondervan. All rights reserved.

Scripture quotations marked (NLT) are taken from the Holy Bible, New Living Translation, Copyright © 1996. Used by permission of Tyndale House Publishers, Inc., Wheaton, Illinois 60189. All rights reserved.

embrace ■ ■ ■
caregiving™

Greetings,

The Bible tells us to accept *one another*, to be kind and compassionate to *one another*, to encourage *one another*, and to instruct *one another*. Also, to live in harmony with *one another*, to love *one another*, to offer hospitality to *one another*, to serve *one another*, and to show mercy and compassion to *one another*. While the phrase *Care for one another* is not specifically stated, I see it as an umbrella statement that covers the many *one another's* and as the basis for biblically based caregiving.

Scripture is a phenomenal source of purpose, direction and inspiration for people taking on the role of caregiver. I wrote this book to help individuals, families, pastors, lay leaders, social service professionals and health care providers understand and apply biblical caregiving principles. I hope to provoke thought and action through the presentation of scripture that relates to the aging and caregiving processes.

When times are tough, as they often are, find comfort in knowing that the Lord has a plan for your life and that He is with you every step of the way. While I was devastated over the illness and death of both my parents while in my mid-thirties, I can look back now and see how God has used my experience for good. Trust that He is doing the same with you. May God's peace be with you!

I invite you to visit www.Caregiving.CC to learn more about Aging America Resources. Our mission is Making Care Easier™ by equipping, empowering and encouraging people to care for one another. We offer articles, books, monthly newsletters and small group curriculum along with input and support for churches and faith-based organizations interested in developing or expanding their care ministry program.

Blessed are the caregivers.

In Christ,

Charles Puchta

embrace ■ ■ ■
caregiving^SM

Embrace caregiving is a service mark of Aging America Resources and is the brand under which we offer our products and services.

Aging America Resources is a 501(c)(3) nonprofit organization.

Comments

When it comes to compassion, scripture is clear: God shows no favoritism. But human beings? Let's be honest ... that's another story. In the church, a legitimate desire to be relevant in order to reach people has become a double-edged sword. Because of the high speed, youth-obsessed culture of the Western world, a simple theological and practical approach to caring for the elderly has been low on our priority scale.

Charles has presented a clear biblical response to this issue. Since God shows no partiality, then this is a long overdue book in our society. I love his mission to equip, encourage and enable people to care for a generation whose voice is often lost in the noise. But above all, this is a book about compassion. And love never fails.

Dave Workman
Pastor and author of *The Outward Focused Life*

Dave Workman is senior pastor of The Vineyard Community Church, which was considered one of the 50 Most Influential Churches in America in 2007 by The Church Report.

Having helped to take care of both my grandparents after my mom's death — and now my father — I am most appreciative of your work and your book. The book offers great points and explanations about the spiritual basis of the kind of loving care our elders deserve.

Rob Portman

> Mr. Portman was recently the director of the Office of Management and Budget serving in President George W. Bush's cabinet. Prior to that, he served as the U.S. Trade Representative and as a Representative of the Second District of Ohio in the United States Congress.

This is a wonderful new book about caregiving. Charles Puchta opens the door to a deeper experience of the spiritual side of caring for one another. This book eloquently addresses the important matter of being present to another human being, while imparting biblical principals.

Charles has given us a valuable and clearly written book to be used by faith community nurses, lay health ministers, clergy, health care professionals and faith community leaders in their practices. This book is filled with insight and wisdom - a truly valuable resource.

Marlene Feagan, MA, BSN, RN, FCN
President, Health Ministries Association, Inc.

> The Health Ministry Association encourages, supports and empowers leaders in the integration of faith and health in their local communities.

Teaching biblical principles of caregiving for aging parents and others should be one of the priorities of the church. In addition to caring for our loved ones, such a study is a great open door for churches to use as an evangelism approach.

Having facilitated the small group curriculum *Caregiving: Caring for Aging Parents* by Charles Puchta, I am more aware of the need and the impact that such a ministry can have.

Charles' new book *Care for One Another* is a valuable resource for preparing to care with the love of Christ for people who may otherwise be overlooked.

Jimmy Ray Lee, D.Min.
President
Living Free/Turning Point Ministries

> Founded in 1988 by Dr. Lee, Living Free provides churches with small group training and focused discipleship curriculums to help people turn to God and His resources when dealing with life's problems.

Charles, I love this book. It was so well written. I love the way you help people relate and explain the scripture so it is relevant to what's happening in our lives. The world is in such turmoil, and people are so confused about themselves, life and even death.

This book helps people understand and apply the various aging and caregiving principles. It is easy to read and best of all based on scripture. The questions at the end of each chapter encourage thought and give people hope for their current situation and the future. No doubt it will be a blessing to a lot of people.

Karen Bankston, PhD, FACHE
Senior Vice President – Drake Center, Inc.

Dr. Bankston serves on the governing council of the American Hospital Association's Section for Long-Term Care & Rehabilitation and was recently named Woman of the Year (Corporate) by the Cincinnati USA Regional Chamber.

This book is dedicated to the many wonderful people
who have been with me along my faith journey
and encouraged me along the way.

Special thanks to my wife Karen, my sister Polly, and
my brother (in-law and in Christ) Gregg.
Your support, love and belief in me are heartfelt.

To our daughters Josie, Ellie and Abbie.
Even though you are only children,
your passion for the Lord and serving others
is already evident in so many ways.

Also, to the Board Members of Aging America
Resources, thanks for your friendship and for
your dedicated service..

CARE *For One Another*

About the Author

Charles Puchta is founder and principal of Aging America Resources (www.Caregiving.CC), Director of the Center for Aging with Dignity (www.SAFEafter60.CC) at the University of Cincinnati College of Nursing and an adjunct instructor for the UC School of Health Services. Puchta is a Certified Senior Advisor, an award-winning author and a nationally recognized authority, advisor, advocate, and speaker on the subject of aging and caregiving.

He has devoted his life to helping individuals, families and professionals anticipate, understand and address the many challenges brought about by aging and illness. His distinctive gift is his ability to take complex subject matter, distill it and communicate it in a way that makes sense to the audience.

Puchta has written numerous books, small group curriculums and other resources addressing aging, health concerns and caregiving issues. He works with churches and faith-based organizations across the country, helping them formulate and implement programs to support the care needs of older adults and caregivers in their community. For more information, visit www.Puchta.CC.

Puchta lives in Loveland, Ohio, with his wife, three daughters and two dogs. A favorite saying, and one that reflects his career and calling is, *"To love what you do and feel that it matters – how could anything be more fun?"*

In addition to the fun he has pursuing his passion, Puchta believes that caregiving should be fulfilling and rewarding for both the care receiver and caregiver. He hopes, and is confident that, this book will provide you with the perspectives and spiritual insight you need to make a difference in the lives of the people with whom you interact.

Contents

1. Biblical Caregiving Principles   19
   - Inspirational Stories
   - God's Promises
2. Aging and Illness   31
   - Person vs. Circumstance
   - Healing and Hope
3. Honor and Obey   45
   - Association Indicates Significance
   - Setting Your Priorities
4. Faith In Action   65
   - Treasures vs. Trust
   - Heavenly Rewards
5. Caregiving Instruction   77
   - Expressing Yourself
   - Set Reasonable Expectations
6. Love and Support   93
   - Forgiveness and Reconciliation
   - Actions vs. Reactions
7. Peace and Purpose   109
   - Living Legacy
   - The Grieving Process
8. Resources and References   123

CARE *For One Another*

1.
Biblical Caregiving Principles

The Bible has a great deal to say about aging and caregiving, and it is filled with practical instruction and helpful perspectives. In this book, I offer a Christian perspective to help you understand and apply biblical caregiving principles. My hope is to encourage people to care for one another with compassion and purpose. I believe if more people provided biblically based care for an aging parent or an ill spouse, the world would be a better place.

Caregiving is almost always more than a person can handle alone. Find guidance, strength and hope through God and His Word. Turn to your Bible and spend quiet time with God on a daily basis. No matter how busy you are, determine to set aside that special time with Him. And remember that He is with you every moment of the day.

> *But joyful are those who have the God of Israel as their helper, whose hope is in the Lord their God. He made heaven and earth, the sea, and everything in them. He keeps every promise forever. He gives justice to the oppressed and food to the hungry. The Lord frees the prisoners. The Lord opens the eyes of the blind. The Lord lifts up those who are weighed down. The Lord loves the godly.* — **Psalm 146:5-8**

Inspirational Stories

Throughout the Bible there are stories that teach us about different aspects of caring for loved ones who are aging and ill. Scripture can help us to understand the aging process and what to anticipate. There are commandments and directives that indicate what is expected of family members and friends. There is also hope for each new day and guidance to help us cope with the unexpected situations and challenges we face.

In the book of Genesis, we read how Joseph honored Jacob, his father, when he became frail. Passages refer to the physical effects of aging and serve as an example of a parent sharing his last request and asking family to honor his wishes upon death. We also read how Jacob's family was at his bedside when he died and how the grieving and mourning process followed death, just as it does today.

The story of Ruth and Naomi paints a picture of love and commitment. After Naomi's husband and two sons died, her daughter-in-law Ruth made incredible sacrifices by staying with Naomi, her mother-in-law, as she traveled back to her homeland. Orpah, the other daughter-in-law chose to return to her family of origin. This passage is significant because it shows that family members respond differently to situations. In today's society in which people are often too busy for their own family, the level of commitment and love Ruth displayed by staying with her mother in-law may seem rather unusual.

As you care for an aging parent or ill spouse, understand that care receivers and caregivers may disagree on the type of care and/or the level of support needed. In some cases, there may not be agreement that care and support are even necessary. Don't be surprised if a loved one denies or is unwilling to talk about health concerns. Avoidance is a coping mechanism.

In the Gospel of Luke (Chapter 10), we find the story of two sisters who had differing styles of caring. The story illustrates how easy it is to become task-oriented and overlook the value of the relationship with the one we are serving. Remember, we are human *beings,* not human *doings.* Often, the time we spend with loved ones is of equal or greater value than anything else we do.

God's Word also teaches us to be realistic about life and death and the effect the aging process has on us all. A recurring theme in the book of Ecclesiastes (verses 12:1-5) is that unless we live life with an eternal perspective, we will not find true joy at any stage of life, especially the Golden Years.

Find comfort knowing that care ministry is close to God's heart, and when you care for one another you are reflecting an aspect of His character to the world, bringing Him glory and pleasure. He will help you in this endeavor, and He wants you to pray to Him for strength, wisdom and resources to accomplish His will.

The Greatest Generation

Older adults are truly America's great generation. Known for their family values and work ethic, they have laid the foundation of prosperity and freedom we enjoy today.

Gray hair is a crown of splendor; it is attained by a righteous life. — **Proverbs 16:31**

What's so special about our elders? Our elders have wisdom from their life experiences. Wisdom comes from years of trial, error and living.

Is not wisdom found among the aged? Does not long life bring understanding? — **Job 12:12**

Though each stage of life presents challenges and opportunities, the benefits of aging are rarely explored and seldom appreciated. Our perspective of aging and older people shapes our view of aging as a blessing or a curse, a privilege or a detriment, or somewhere in between. Growing old and maintaining a desirable quality of life is truly a gift.

Older adults enjoy growth and development opportunities that are equal in value to those of younger people and that should be respected. The tapestry of life for older adults reflects a richness that comes only from years of experience. We can learn valuable lessons in life from older generations. We should treat our elders with dignity and honor.

Don't get frustrated by the little things our aging loved ones may do or say. Instead, recognize the many ways God made your parents special. Cherish their wit and wisdom and be thankful that you have a parent or loved one to enjoy.

Respecting your elders is not just something your mother told you to do; it is something that God has instructed us to do. Showing respect to older generations also models a behavior and teaches younger generations how to respect older adults and eventually how to treat you.

I encourage families and faith-based organizations to advocate for older adults and seek their involvement. Don't set older adults aside and lead them to believe that their lives and opinions don't count. Everyone has the potential to live life, to make a difference, and to bring glory to God to the very end.

> *I eagerly expect and hope that I will in no way be ashamed, but will have sufficient courage so that now as always Christ will be exalted in my body, whether by life or by death.* — **Philippians 1: 20**

Older adults often have time, talent and treasure that can benefit you and your community. Are you recognizing the older adults in your life for their wisdom and experience? Or are you trying to find places to put older adults and get them out of the way?

Instead of isolating them, we should involve older adults and integrate them throughout our lives, our churches and our communities. Consider ways to engage them and leverage their skills, abilities and interests. God's Word makes it clear that a person is never too old to do God's work.

The gray-haired and the aged are on our side, ...
— **Job 15:10a**

They will still bear fruit in old age, ...
— **Psalm 92:14a**

Everyone has a powerful desire to feel wanted, useful, loved and appreciated. Everyone longs to be significant in the lives of other people, especially family and friends. When we feel unwanted or unimportant, we may try to give the impression that it doesn't bother us even though we feel heartbroken. The pain of rejection can shatter the core of a person's identity and being.

In the book *The Angry Man*, Stephen Arterburn and David Stoop write, *"Identity is a matter of character, not accomplishment, a matter of being and relating, not doing."*

Delving Deeper

People tend to be familiar with Bible verses such as *honor your father and mother* (Exodus 20:12a) and *do to others, what you would have them do to you,* (Matthew 7:12.) However, many have not delved into these passages with the same fervor as scripture that provides daily hope and encouragement or that is directly related to the trials and tribulations of everyday life. Throughout this book, we will delve deeper and explore scripture to understand its lessons and identify biblical caregiving principles that we can apply to our lives.

As you seek God's guidance and direction, remember that the Bible is a love letter offering hope, peace and purpose to those who seek and follow the Lord. Turn to God and His Word on a daily basis for strength, direction and encouragement.

> NOTE: *As you study the Bible, you will certainly find many more references to each topic discussed in this book. In selecting scripture, I made a concerted effort to include passages that offer unique perspectives as opposed to sharing multiple passages that emphasize the same point.*

God's Promises

God never promised us days without pain, laughter without sorrow, or sun without rain; but He did promise strength to get through each day, comfort for the tears, and light for the way. As you provide care and support for a parent, spouse, sibling, relative or friend, turn to God for strength and hope.

The LORD gives strength to his people; the Lord blesses his people with peace. — **Psalm 29:11**

May God's peace be with you. As you try to make sense of the challenges you face, know that our Lord is sovereign. Trust in God!

Trust in the LORD with all your heart and lean not on your own understanding. — **Proverbs 3:5**

Regardless of your situation, have faith. God knows what you are going through, and He uses all situations for good.

And we know that in all things God works for the good of those who love him... — **Romans 8:28a**

Bill Hybels, senior pastor of Willow Creek Community Church, writes in his book *Who Are You When No One's Looking*, "Does your problem seem bigger than life, bigger than God himself? It isn't. God is infinitely bigger than any problem you ever had or will have, and every time you call a problem unsolvable, you mock God. With God all things are possible."

Rejoice in the Lord always. I will say it again: Rejoice! Let your gentleness be evident to all. The Lord is near. Do not be anxious about anything, but in everything, by prayer and petition, with thanksgiving, present your requests to God. And the peace of God, which transcends all understanding, will guard your hearts and your minds in Christ Jesus. — **Philippians 4:4-7**

Blessings

For many people, our lives have become so routine that we take things for granted. A bump in the road can be a necessary wake-up call to get us to stop and reflect on the many ways we are blessed each and every day. One of those blessings is our health.

Often it is when we experience ongoing pain or end up in the hospital that we recognize the truly precious gift of good health. Take a minute and consider the complexity of the human body and what a miracle life really is.

As a caregiver, take steps now to preserve your own health by improving your diet, reducing stress, and exercising regularly. Those of us who do not take time to tend to our health and engage in wellness activities now will certainly have to make time for illness later. Maintaining your mental, physical and spiritual health is critical. If your health is compromised, you will be unable to effectively care for one another.

> *This is the day the LORD has made; let us rejoice and be glad in it.* — **Psalm 118:24**

Each and every day, give thanks to the Lord for life. After all, your body is your earthly home and is a gift from God. There is a lot of truth in the saying *"You can't put a price on good health."* Our health becomes a cornerstone to everything we do each day.

The Bible Has The Answers!

The Bible is truly awesome! I am continually amazed at how everything imaginable is addressed in it.

> *For the word of God is living and active.*
> — **Hebrews 4:12a**

One thing that sets Christian caregiving apart is that, as Christians, we depend upon God's guidance and direction in our helping ministry. Anyone can learn facts and helping methods, but without sensitivity to the Holy Spirit's guidance there is a lack of purpose and hope. God alone knows the deepest needs of His people, and He can help us understand how best to care for loved ones, even when they do not openly express their need or desire for assistance.

Reflection and Discussion

Are there certain passages from the Bible that you turn to for strength and encouragement? What are they?

What are a few of the health and care issues that you are most concerned about or that are most challenging?

Do you believe that understanding and applying biblical caregiving principles provides an advantage to you as you care for one another? Why? Why not?

KEY LEARNINGS – *Top three findings from this chapter:*

1.
2.
3.

ACTION ITEMS - *Things you want to do or do differently:*

Check when Completed	*Action Item*	*Target Completion Date*

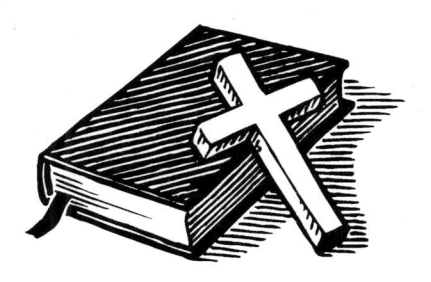

Prayer

Dear Heavenly Father, help me to be faithful to that which You have called me to do, and help me to fully recognize that calling in my life. Help me to unselfishly love my parents (or spouse, relative or friend) and support them during their (his/her) times of need. Help me Lord to honor them (him/her) in every way. Please fill me with Your Spirit, Lord, so that love, gentleness, kindness and patience are ever present in my life. In Jesus' precious and holy name. Amen.

Biblical Caregiving Principles

2.
Aging and Illness

Human life has a natural cycle that has existed since the time of Adam and Eve. Aging and death were not the design of God's original creation but have become part of the natural rhythm of life as we know it.

Then the LORD said, "My Spirit will not contend with man forever, for he is mortal; his days will be a hundred and twenty years." — **Genesis 6:3**

Aging is a process of gradual change over time that is most noticeable in children and older adults. We reach our peak physical functioning and ability in our 20's and early 30's. These are the years that our bodies are the strongest, our senses are the keenest, and our minds are the sharpest.

Remember your Creator in the days of your youth, before the days of trouble come and the years approach when you will say, "I find no pleasure in them."
— **Ecclesiastes 12:1**

God's Word teaches us to be realistic about life and death and the impact the aging process has upon us all. While the sequence of age-related change is similar, the rate at which we experience change tends to be quite individual, often based on lifestyle choices, genetics and environmental factors.

While aging is a fact of life, I believe the idea of normal or successful aging is being able to do all that you want to without being limited by disease, a lack of energy, or a lack of financial resources.

The term *"successful aging"* first appeared in professional literature in 1961 in the inaugural issue of The Gerontologist. While much has been written about the concept of successful aging since then, there is not a single universally adopted or accepted definition of successful aging. A problem using the term successful is that people who are facing challenges and limitations might view their aging as failure.

As part of a study published in the Journal of the American Geriatrics Society, people aged 65 and older identified what they believed were characteristics of normal or successful aging. Here is what they indicated:

Being able to...
- Take care of myself until close to the time of my death
- Make choices about things that affect how I age, like my diet, exercise and smoking
- Cope with the challenges of my later years
- Act according to my own inner standards and values
- Meet all of my needs and some of my wants
- Successfully manage chronic disease(s)
- Have friends and family who are there for me
- Feel good about myself
- Feel satisfied with my life the majority of the time
- Stay involved with the world and people around me
- Adjust to changes related to aging
- Not feel lonely or isolated.

I believe these findings are significant in light of the many indignities people face with age. Growing old and maintaining functional abilities and a desirable quality of life is truly a gift. According to the Administration on Aging (Profile of Older Adults: 2008), over 40% of older adults reported difficulties with activities of daily living associated with independent living, and 28% struggle with personal care activities such as bathing, hygiene, dressing and more.

Older adults face increased risk for illnesses such as arthritis, Alzheimer's, cancer, heart disease, Parkinson's and stroke. And when people encounter disease and face limitations, many have a difficult time accepting their situation and accepting help.

Throughout the Bible, we read of the effects of the aging process. I find that many Americans have an overly optimistic outlook for the Golden Years, when the fact of the matter is that approximately 80% of older adults are living with at least one chronic illness. While many chronic illnesses can be successfully managed by making lifestyle modifications and with medication, illnesses often limit peoples' ability to perform everyday activities.

Let's look at what the Bible tells us about the effects of aging and disease by looking at six specific passages.

1. *Now Israel's eyes were failing because of old age, and he could hardly see.* — **Genesis 48:10a**

    As we age, the pupil of the eye becomes less responsive to changes in lighting, making it difficult to see in the dark. Also, the lens of the eye gradually thickens and yellows and there is a loss in visual acuity, which is the ability to notice detail. Diseases of the eye such as cataracts, diabetic retinopathy, glaucoma and macular degeneration also affect a person's ability to see.

Aging and Illness

2. *When King David was old and well advanced in years, he could not keep warm even when they put covers over him.*
   — 1 Kings 1:1

   As a result of lower body weight, inactivity, reduced muscle mass and changes to the skin, many older adults are more sensitive to air temperature and are less insulated from the cold.

3. *In his old age, however, his feet became diseased.*
   — 1 Kings 15:23

   As we age we are more susceptible to becoming diabetic. People with diabetes and other diseases that affect circulation are prone to foot problems.

4. *My flesh and my heart may fail, but God is the strength of my heart and my portion forever.*
   — Psalm 73:26

   Heart disease is the second-leading cause of death for people age 65 and older. It is the leading cause of death for people age 75 and older.

5. *... he had a stroke, and he lay paralyzed on his bed like a stone.* **— 1 Samuel 25:37b (NLT)**

   Stroke is the third-leading cause of death in America and the No. 1 cause of adult disability?

6. *Remember him before your legs — the guards of your house — start to tremble; and before your shoulders — the strong men — stoop. Remember him before your teeth — your few remaining servants — stop grinding; ...*
   — Ecclesiastes 12:3a (NLT)

Once we reach the age of 30, bone marrow gradually starts to disappear from the bones in our arms and legs, and there is a reduction in calcium that leads to decreased bone mass? As a result, older adults may be frail and have brittle bones. Also, our teeth become more sensitive to hot and cold temperatures. Tooth decay, gum disease and discoloration are common concerns regardless of age.

Facing Illness

Informing people that they have a life-changing or life-threatening disease is often associated with *"dropping the bomb."* After a diagnosis is shared, it is then up to each individual and his or her family to sort through the rubble and pick up the pieces.

> *So do not fear, for I am with you; do not be dismayed, for I am your God. I will strengthen you and help you; I will uphold you with my righteous right hand.* — **Isaiah 41:10**

Receiving any diagnosis can be a life-altering experience in which people may face both a sense of relief and fear. Relief often comes from placing a name on signs and symptoms, and developing a treatment plan to address the illness. Simultaneously, fear often emerges due to the uncertainty of the future with a chronic, debilitating or terminal disease.

In one of his devotionals, Patrick Morley writes, *"Some illnesses are routine and short, like colds and flu. One illness, morning sickness, is even a sign of joy. But other diseases — like cancer — are terrifying and may cause disability, infirmity and death."*

Whether it is when a diagnosis is made or any time throughout the disease process, it is common for people to:

- Cry out to God and ask why
- Rely more on flesh than faith
- Get frustrated
- Overdo it
- Try to control aspects of life.

At times, you may not understand why you and your family are facing these challenges, but if you seek God, you will find Him. God promises to hear our prayers and meet our needs. Keep in mind that His meeting your needs may be inconsistent with the way you might want your prayers to be answered. As the saying goes, hindsight is 20/20. While you may not be clear how God is working in your life, over time He will reveal His plan to you if you seek Him.

There is a time for everything, and a season for every activity under heaven:
A time to be born and a time to die,
A time to plant and a time to uproot,
A time to kill and a time to heal,
A time to tear down and a time to build,
A time to weep and a time to laugh,
A time to mourn and a time to dance,
— **Ecclesiastes 3:1-4**

Just as winter, spring, summer and fall come and go, we face seasons in life that are filled with challenges. Know that a season is not a brief time, but a limited time. No season lasts forever. So why do we experience seasons? I believe that seasons signify the following:

- A time to experience God
- A time to refocus on God
- A time to learn from God
- A time to grow in God.

While we sometimes wish we could be in quick mode rather than the more patient slow mode, there is a purpose for every season of life. Also, just as we tend to have a favorite season and one that is our least favorite, there are seasons that we go through that are necessary for us to enjoy the seasons to come. So whatever the harsh conditions of one season, trust in God and know that he uses all things for good.

When a loved one becomes ill, in addition to understanding the diagnosis, give consideration to the prognosis and how an illness or disease is likely to affect day-to-day living activities. With some medical conditions such as arthritis and stroke, limitations may be apparent. But with dementia, diabetes and other conditions, a person's limitations may be less obvious.

Regardless of whether limitations are obvious or not, know that many people may be resistant to accepting care and support from family and friends because they do not want to be a burden. For the care process to be optimal, there needs to be recognition, participation and acceptance of both the care receiver and caregiver(s).

Person vs. Circumstances

When a loved one is diagnosed with a medical condition, family and friends tend to treat the person differently, whether knowingly or not. Family and friends may be afraid of a disease like cancer or be reluctant to acknowledge a disease because, as humans, we struggle to accept our own mortality.

Regardless of whether or not we choose to face the reality of a disease, many people are afraid to ask a person about his or her health. Avoiding conversation because you are not sure what to say or ask tends to create tension and cause people to feel awkward.

To help relate to loved ones, make sure to distinguish between the person and the circumstances. Treat the person the same as before he or she had a disease or disability. For example, if a person becomes hard of hearing, don't ignore him or her. Instead, treat the person as before and control the circumstances; turn off a TV or radio playing in the background or go to a room with less noise. Face the person, get closer to one another, speak a bit louder and enunciate your words.

If a disease causes you to feel uncomfortable or awkward, you might find it helpful to replace the name of the disease (e.g. cancer, heart disease, Parkinson's, ALS) with the words "*broken leg.*" Why? Because it will help you interact with the person without feeling awkward. Go ahead. Try it. Chances are you will treat the person more like you did before he or she was diagnosed. Imagine the person has a broken leg instead of a disease ...

- What would you say to him or her?
- What questions would you ask?
- What type of assistance would you provide?

You see, we tend not to be afraid of a broken leg like we often are of disease. For example, if a person has a broken leg, it is common for family and friends to ask...

- What happened?
- When did it happen?
- Are you in pain?
- How do you feel?
- What can I do to help?

Over time chances are people will inquire about what to expect. For example ...

- When do you get the cast off?
- Are you able to drive?

- Are you going to need rehabilitation?
- How is the recovery process going?
- What long-term effects might this have on your ability to _____ (e.g. climb stairs, go grocery shopping, play golf).

Whether a person has a broken leg or a life-changing or life-threatening disease, ask questions and acknowledge the medical condition. Chances are everyone will be more comfortable. The alternative is that there is a huge white elephant in the room that no one is willing to acknowledge, yet everyone knows is there.

Also, don't assume you know how aging or illness is affecting a loved one, or what he or she wants, needs or is feeling. Instead, talk and ask open-ended questions that can help uncover concerns and face the realities of the situation. Know that some people may be reluctant to share their concerns, and be sensitive and observant as you try to figure out how you can best provide support and encouragement. Do whatever you can to keep the lines of communication open.

Do not cast me away when I am old; do not forsake me when my strength is gone. — **Psalm 71:9**

Even when I am old and gray, do not forsake me, ...
— **Psalm 71:18a**

If, as result of aging, a loved one finds everyday life to be increasingly challenging, pray to God to strengthen, guide and protect both the care receiver (*your loved one*) and the caregivers (*you, other family members and friends*). If disease strikes, lift your petitions for healing, strength and comfort to God. Pray over loved ones in the name of Jesus and claim victory by His shed blood. Pray for total and complete healing.

Healing and Hope

Throughout the Gospels, there are numerous stories of healing. As I read about the various encounters, what stands out to me is that the people seeking healing all had incredible faith. They believed Jesus would and could heal them of their diseases. For example:

> *Jesus went throughout Galilee, teaching in their synagogues, preaching the good news of the kingdom, and healing every disease and sickness among the people. News about him spread all over Syria, and people brought to him all who were ill with various diseases, those suffering severe pain, the demon-possessed, those having seizures, and the paralyzed, and he healed them.*
> — **Matthew 4:23-24**

> *A man with leprosy came and knelt before him and said, "Lord, if you are willing, you can make me clean." Jesus reached out his hand and touched the man. "I am willing," he said. "Be clean!" Immediately he was cured of his leprosy.* — **Matthew 8:2-3**

> *When Jesus had entered Capernaum, a centurion came to him, asking for help. "Lord," he said, "my servant lies at home paralyzed and in terrible suffering." Jesus said to him, "I will go and heal him." The centurion replied, "Lord, I do not deserve to have you come under my roof. But just say the word, and my servant will be healed. For I myself am a man under authority, with soldiers under me. I tell this one, 'Go,' and he goes; and that one, 'Come,' and he comes. I say to my servant, 'Do this,' and he does it." When Jesus heard this, he was astonished and said to those following him, "I tell you the truth, I have not found anyone in Israel with such great faith. Then Jesus said to*

the centurion, "Go! It will be done just as you believed it would." And his servant was healed at that very hour.
— **Matthew 8:5-10, 13**

When Jesus came into Peter's house, he saw Peter's mother-in-law lying in bed with a fever. He touched her hand and the fever left her, and she got up and began to wait on him. — **Matthew 8:14-15**

Some men brought to him a paralytic, lying on a mat. When Jesus saw their faith, he said to the paralytic, "Take heart, son; your sins are forgiven."
— **Matthew 9:2**

Did you notice how the stories in the Gospel of Matthew reflect many scenarios and different types of disease? Jesus healed by touching people and by being touched. He healed people at the request of others. And, He gives us authority over sickness and disease as well.

Do you believe in the power of healing, healing prayer and healing touch? Based on denominational affiliation, many people are not comfortable praying over a loved one or anointing a person with oil. If you want to claim victory over disease and pray for healing, and would like someone to stand with you, talk to others within your faith-based community for direction and support.

Reflection and Discussion

Carefully consider and list any health-related problems that are currently affecting you and your family.

Are there certain resources (e.g. books, organizations or websites) that you have found to be helpful that you might share with others?

Are there certain prayers or encouraging words that others might find helpful?

What are your thoughts about healing touch and healing prayer? If that is something you are interested in exploring, who might you contact for support?

KEY LEARNINGS – *Top three findings from this chapter:*

1.

2.

3.

ACTION ITEMS - *Things you want to do or do differently:*

Check when Completed	Action Item	Target Completion Date

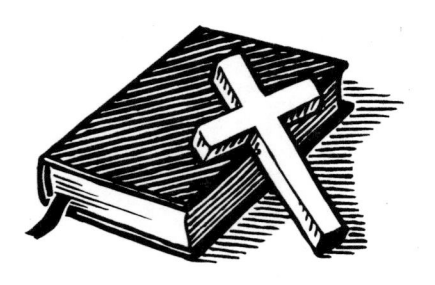

Prayer

Lord God, I come before you with a humble heart. I place my trust in you Lord. I pray for total and complete healing of (insert name). Lord God you are my everything. Without you I am nothing. Forgive me Lord of my sins and help me to repent. Thank you Lord for your promises. Thank you Lord for the gift of peace that is beyond understanding. Thank you Lord for healing. Help me Lord to believe and to achieve. By the shed blood of Jesus, I claim victory over disease and distress. In Your name I pray. Amen.

3.
Honor and Obey

In the second book of the Bible, we see the first reference to honoring your father and mother. As people read the Fifth Commandment, I believe there are certain words that tend to roll off the tongue without much consideration to the meaning. These words are: *honor, so that,* and *live long.*

> *Honor your father and your mother, so that you may live long in the land the Lord your God is giving you.*
> **— Exodus 20:12**

It's About Honor

To understand what the word *honor* means, let's review the definition. Webster's Dictionary uses the words *"high respect; esteem; glory or recognition; distinction; high rank; great privilege"* to define honor. Notice how the word honor is always positive and privileged.

Honor is commonly associated with people who have achieved a position of significance. For example, *Your Honor* when referring to a judge, or the *Honor Roll* at school referring to students whose academic performance merits recognition.

If you think of honoring someone, what is involved? I believe that if we were recognizing someone such as a former president, celebrity or professional athlete, the person who is being honored would most likely be...

- The center of attention.
- Someone you want to be near (e.g. sitting at the same table with, getting your picture taken with).
- A person you would want to talk with, learn from, ask questions to, and hear his or her story.
- Someone you would tell your friends about and be proud of knowing.

Are the attributes of honor listed above consistent with how you honor your parents? Or, is your relationship better described as insignificant or "out of sight, out of mind?"

Consider this: God predestined each one of us. God chose our parents, and while it may not be apparent at the time, He uses all things for good. Honoring your mother and father is a commandment, not a choice or suggestion, and it is for our own good.

> *...and to observe the Lord's commands and decrees I am giving you today for your own good?*
> — **Deuteronomy 10:13**

While every family has issues, a phrase I occasionally hear is *"You can pick your friends, but you can't pick your family."* If you come from what may be described as a dysfunctional family and your relationships are strained or damaged, honoring your father and mother may be difficult; however, I have not read anything in the Bible that indicates any exceptions.

If your family relationships are best described as non-existent or challenged, spend time in prayer asking the Lord for strength, guidance and direction about how to reconcile. It seems we are often creatures of habit. We know how our loved ones are going to react before a situation occurs. Surprising someone with a loving gesture he or she does not expect may help to begin mending broken relationships and honor your parents in a way that is pleasing to God.

> *If you have unresolved family of origin issues where there may have been physical, sexual or emotional abuse, I encourage you to seek counseling to address and work through your issues.*

It is difficult for some people to differentiate between honoring their parents and enabling their parents. Finding the right balance between helping someone and encouraging them to help themselves can be challenging. The tendency is to want to be compassionate and help make life easier, especially for someone who is aging or ill.

However, when we do doing things for people they could do themselves, we run the risk of enabling. It may become necessary to establish expectations and set boundaries. Doing so can help you honor your parents while managing your own life.

As you reflect on the word *honor,* consider ways you can honor your parents, such as being involved in their life, involving them in your life and seeking their input and advice on major life decisions.

Another way to honor your parents is to pray for them regularly. Ask God to comfort your parents and relieve them of their fears or anything else that may be robbing them of joy. Also, pray that God will shine a bright light on the path for you, bring clarity to your role as a family caregiver, and give you insight to the issue(s) underlying your parent's actions or inactions.

Why Honor

Just after we are commanded to *honor*, we are told why. It is important to note that the words *so that* are conditional. Notice that the Fifth Commandment is the first one with a promise. In other words, *if* you honor, *then* you will receive.

> *Honor your father and your mother, so that you may live long in the land the Lord your God is giving you.*
> **— Exodus 20:12**

God offers his people abundant life filled with joy, peace and purpose. When the Bible states that you will *live long*, this is not a guarantee of longevity in terms of chronological age. While you may be blessed with longevity, the real benefit is truly being able to live. That is to live a blessed life, free from the bondage of purposeful sin, stress and guilt that many people encounter. More importantly, by honoring our parents, we ultimately honor God. Are you living an abundant life free from guilt, shame and busyness?

Association Indicates Significance

You have probably heard the cliché of being able to tell the character of a man by the company he keeps. I believe that the same concept applies to understanding the importance God places on the Fifth Commandment. Right along with the commandment of honoring our parents we find the commandments:

- *You shall have no other gods before me.*
- *You shall not make for yourself an idol.*
- *You shall not misuse the name of the Lord your God.*

- *You shall not murder.*
- *You shall not commit adultery.*
- *You shall not steal.*
- *You shall not give false testimony against your neighbor.*
- *You shall not covet.*

Note that seven of the Ten Commandments specifically tell us things we must NOT do. The first commandment is also similar in that it states *Thou shalt have* NO *other gods before me.* The only commandments that tell us what we MUST do are the fourth and fifth.

- *Remember the Sabbath day by keeping it holy.*
- *Honor your father and your mother.*

I find it amazing to think that God's Top 10 includes instruction on how we should respect and love our parents. With all the children and teenagers who are struggling, trying to fit in and seeking purpose in their lives, I might have expected one of the Ten Commandments to say something like *Cherish your children raising them in a way that is pleasing to God.*

Also, are you aware that the Fourth Commandment is about rest? People who take on the role of caregiver must achieve balance between fulfilling responsibilities and rejuvenating the spirit, soul and body. Sabbath is a Hebrew word meaning to cease or desist. It is a day that is given to rest and remember God so that our bodies, souls and spirits can be refreshed. It is a reminder of the eternal rest God has promised his people. Yes, God wants us to rest and replenish ourselves. He wants us to take a day off every week. If you have always thought that the Fourth Commandment was about going to church on the seventh day, read the following passages: Exodus 20:8-11 and Exodus 16:21-30.

By the seventh day God had finished the work he had been doing; so on the seventh day he rested from all his work. And God blessed the seventh day and made it holy, because on it he rested from all the work of creating that he had done. — **Genesis 2:2-3**

In the book of Genesis, God is establishing order in His creation; and as part of that order, He makes the seventh day holy (*set apart especially for Him*). A time of rest is incorporated into the natural fabric of creation.

Six days you shall labor, but on the seventh day you shall rest; even during the plowing season and harvest you must rest. — **Exodus 34:21**

The Exodus passage makes it clear that whatever may appear to be necessary or urgent can and should wait so that we take time to replenish ourselves, thus avoid getting burned out. The same principle applies to caregiving. Caregivers are often driven by many needs that keep us from taking care of our responsibilities to God and ourselves. It is okay to ask for help and to make arrangements for others to participate in the caregiving process. While we don't want to overlook someone's needs, we do need our rest.

Repetition Reinforces the Point

We first learn about the consequences of failing to honor our parents in the book of Deuteronomy. The consequences are reinforced and referenced numerous times throughout the Bible.

Cursed is the man who dishonors his father or his mother.
— **Deuteronomy 27:16a**

> *For God said, 'Honor your father and mother' and 'Anyone who curses his father or mother must be put to death.'*
> — **Matthew 15:4**

Being cursed is the opposite of being blessed. Just as blessings are the reward for being obedient, curses are the consequence of disobedience. It means that our sin and disobedience separates us from God. In other words our sins of omission (*the things we do not do that we should*) and commission (*the things we do that we shouldn't*) both bring consequences. Rebelling against God and forfeiting the gifts of abundant life, His blessings and love, is truly a sacrifice.

The word blessing leads many people to think of the book *Prayer of Jabez*. In this book, author Bruce Wilkinson shares with us God's desire to pour out His blessing on us. Think about how much God loves each and every one of us. He loves us more than we will ever comprehend. Consider how disappointing and foolish it is to dishonor our parents and turn our back to God.

> *... so that Christ may dwell in your hearts through faith. And I pray that you, being rooted and established in love, may have power, together with all the saints, to grasp how wide and long and high and deep is the love of Christ, and to know this love that surpasses knowledge — that you may be filled to the measure of all the fullness of God.*
> — **Ephesians 3:17-19**

Clarification on Honoring

As parents become less quick-witted, slower in pace, stubborn or independent, it is easy to be frustrated or impatient with them. Passages from the books of Matthew and Proverbs tell of appropriate behavior when our parents age.

Honor your father and mother, and love your neighbor as yourself. — **Matthew 19:19**

Listen to your father, who gave you life, and do not despise your mother when she is old. — **Proverbs 23:22**

Most people have heard and thought about what it means to *Love your neighbor as yourself;* however, the Proverbs passage is less known. The idea of listening to your father suggests wisdom and experience — father knows best. The second part of the passage specifically instructs us what not to do: *do not despise your mother when she is old.* I might have expected something more like, be patient, loving and kind with your mother as she ages. But the point is more clearly stated by using a negative to insinuate a positive. It is as though a normal reaction would be to get frustrated with our mother and therefore, we need to be told not to become irritated or annoyed with her.

Know that honoring our parents is not only the right thing to do; it is something that God has commanded. The word Commandment indicates authority or law.

Setting Your Priorities

Honoring is done with a sincere heart. Genuine honor from the heart is not just an obligation. When something is an obligation, it becomes a chore instead of a joy.

I rarely hear people say *"I have so much free time, let me know what I can do to help."* Instead what I hear is *"I'll try to squeeze you in next week"* or *"How about we get together next month."* Although our lives are busy, have you noticed that people tend to find time for the things they enjoy? Likewise, people tend to make excuses to avoid doing the things they do not enjoy or do not want to do.

Who among us will not make the time for the things that are truly important to us? God clearly tells us that our family and home should be priorities.

Are your parents a priority in your life? Do you prioritize them into your schedule or do you try to fit them in here and there? To truly honor your father and mother, they should be a priority in your life. Whether it is talking with them on the telephone a few times each week, or seeing them in person on a regular basis, having some level of regular contact is consistent with the expectation of honor.

When I think of the saying *"Altitude is a reflection of Attitude,"* I think of it in a heavenly sense. That is, the better our attitude about the situations and challenges we face, the easier it is to be more Christ-like and enjoy the gift of abundant life. Jesus never turned away at the sight of lepers. He never spoke out against those who flogged and crucified him. Rather he accepted and loved them and He prayed for them. In fact, he tells us that if someone hits us on one cheek, we should turn and offer up the other. Even though for many people family relationships are anything but perfect, our responsibility to honor remains the same.

Obedience and the Golden Rule

As children, many of us where taught to obey our parents, and to follow the Golden Rule. In this section we delve into the meaning of each phrase.

To understand what it means to obey, we need to start by distinguishing between the concepts of obedience and accountability.

- Obedience is complying with God's desires, wishes and commands for our lives.

- Accountability is bearing the responsibility of obeying. We are ultimately accountable or responsible to God for everything we do in life, including obeying our parents and thus pleasing the Lord.

Children, obey your parents in everything, for this pleases the Lord. — **Colossians 3:19-21**

Adult children tend to feel challenged when their offers of assistance or helpful suggestions are rejected by parents. If your parents do not agree with you or accept your offers of care and support, do you simply give in and do as they request?

Questions I often hear include, *"But what if I don't agree with them?"* and *"What if they are just plain wrong?"* After all, Colossians says *Obey your parents in everything.* To answer these questions, you may need to ponder the following questions to help you determine what to do.

- Are your parents rational, of sound mind and able to make informed decisions?

- Does it appear your parents have sufficient information and understanding of the likely consequences?

- Might your parents be acting out of fear such as the fear of change, the fear of the unknown, the fear of the inability to cope, etc?

- What are the risks if you do nothing and do not challenge your parent or even forcefully push your opinion? Are your parents and other people at risk of injury?

As you consider the choices loved ones are making, it is important to help people distinguish between *needs* and *wants*. People often get so caught up and focused on what they want, they overlook the needs of their loved ones.

- Needs are things that are critically important to one's health, well being and safety.

- Wants are the *"nice to haves."* Often, these are things to which people have become accustomed.

How can you tell if something is a need or a want? One simple way is to listen to what someone says. For example, "*I want ...* " Change can be hard for anyone, especially an older person. If you believe that your parent's health needs are not adequately being met, it may be necessary to take action. Older people may be unaware or unwilling to accept what might be best for them. Older adults can also be set in their ways and resistant to change.

Words that are often associated with older people include independent, proud and stubborn. Many older people have been self-sufficient all their lives and may want to do things their way and without assistance. Some will even attempt to hide their challenges and limitations because they don't want the family to get involved.

It is important to understand and consider what might happen if you do not challenge your parents. For example, what if mom or dad should fall and not be able to summon help? What is the possibility of a parent leaving the stove on and causing a fire? What if you have concerns for a parent's driving and his or her ability to react to an unexpected situation?

Example of Obedience

When I speak of obeying our parents, I am referring to honoring their expressed wishes and desires. The call to obey is different when the person is a minor (*younger than 18*) versus someone who is considered an adult. While minor children are under the authority of their parents, adult children are free to make their own choices regardless of what parents may suggest.

As adults, we honor our parents by obeying their wishes for themselves. I believe we are called to carry out our loved one's wishes and not impose or force our desires on them. In the first book of the Bible, we see an example of an adult child obeying his father and carrying out his father's wishes.

> *When the time drew near for Israel to die, he called for his son Joseph and said to him, "If I have found favor in your eyes, put your hand under my thigh and promise that you will show me kindness and faithfulness. Do not bury me in Egypt, but when I rest with my fathers, carry me out of Egypt and bury me where they are buried." "I will do as you say," he said. "Swear to me," he said. Then Joseph swore to him, and Israel worshiped as he leaned on the top of his staff.* — **Genesis 47:29-31**

> *Then he gave them these instructions: "I am about to be gathered to my people. Bury me with my fathers in the cave in the field of Ephron the Hittite, the cave in the field of Machpelah, near Mamre in Canaan, which Abraham bought as a burial place from Ephron the Hittite, along with the field. There Abraham and his wife Sarah were buried, there Isaac and his wife Rebekah were buried, and there I buried Leah. The field and the cave in it were bought from the Hittites. When Jacob had finished giving*

instructions to his sons, he drew his feet up into the bed, breathed his last and was gathered to his people.
— **Genesis 49:29-33**

Obedience and Honor

As parents age and become more dependent, we need to apply all the lessons we have learned from the Bible and throughout life to help us discern what is best or right for each particular situation. While we are commanded to obey our parents, we know that God has the ultimate authority over our lives and we are called to obey His Word.

As you care for your parents, what you believe to be in their best interest may be inconsistent with their desires or preferences. It may mean making tough decisions against their wishes. For example, if a parent is neglecting him or herself it may be necessary to intervene. Self-neglect refers to the failure of an adult to provide for him or herself so as to avoid physical harm or mental anguish. It includes the failure of the person to provide for his or her basic daily needs (*e.g. cleanliness of living quarters*) and self-care (*e.g. eating, bathing.*)

Always keep your parents' best interests in mind and do not let your own wants get in the way of their needs. Should you feel it necessary to intervene and make a decision that contradicts your parents, you will know in your heart if your motivation is pure and honorable. Remember, God knows our thoughts and our hearts better than we do, so be honest with yourself when examining your motives.

In John 9:23, we see an example where a parent defers to a grown child to speak for himself. The passage states, *He is of age, ask him.* Once a person reaches a certain age, they are expected to make their own decisions. If you believe that your parent is not making rational decisions, consider the risks of doing nothing to intervene. Where is the greater risk or danger? God does not want us to enable our parents to endanger themselves or anyone around them. Consider the greater good. The combination of matching a person's needs with the available options is something about which you will want to pray. Let God provide the guidance and direction that helps you to make the best informed decision that ultimately honors and obeys both your parent and Him.

> *If you are a caregiver, know that the care recipient has the right and responsibility to make all decisions, as long as he or she has the mental capacity to do so. You may not agree with a decision, but it does not mean you should step in and take over. Just as we have all had the freedom to make choices in our lives, our parents also have the right to make choices. I believe when people make poor choices they often lack knowledge and are unaware of the consequences of their actions or inactions.*

Respecting our Elders

The effects of aging may be inevitable, but these do not lessen a person's value. In contemporary Western culture, the young are considered more valuable than the elderly. This is not the case in every society, nor has it always been this way in our culture. The following verses appear to be more consistent with many Middle Eastern cultures and African-American cultures where older adults are more highly revered and valued.

> *'Rise in the presence of the aged, show respect for the elderly and revere your God. I am the Lord'*
> — **Leviticus 19:32**

> *Do not rebuke an older man harshly, but exhort him as if he were your father.* — **1 Timothy 5:1**

Honor and Obey

Most of us have been told to respect our elders since we were children. What does it mean to respect our elders? It may be easier to understand the meaning and application of the word respect by first looking at the word disrespect.

Disrespect includes things such as ignoring someone's thoughts or feelings, being condescending, being neglectful, forcing your opinion, or being rude or selfish. Now consider the opposites. There is a strong connection between the words honor, obey and respect. I think of The Golden Rule. *Do unto others as you would have them do to you.* — Luke 6:31. Isn't that really what it is all about? *The Wooden Bowl* story clearly makes the point.

The Wooden Bowl

A frail old man went to live with his son, daughter-in-law and 4-year-old grandson. The old man's hands trembled, his eyesight blurred, and his step faltered. The family ate together at the table, but the elderly grandfather's shaky hands and failing sight made eating difficult. Peas rolled off the spoon onto the floor. When he grasped the glass, milk spilled on the tablecloth. The son and daughter-in-law became irritated with the mess. "We must do something with grandpa," said the son. "I have had enough of spilled milk, noisy eating, and food on the floor." So the husband and the wife set a small table in the corner.

There grandpa ate alone while the rest of the family enjoyed their dinner. Since Grandpa had broken a dish or two, his food was served in a wooden bowl. When the family glanced in Grandpa's direction, sometimes he had a tear in his eye as he sat alone. Still the only words the couple had for him were sharp admonitions when he dropped his fork or spilled food. The 4-year-old watched it all in silence.

One evening before supper, the father noticed his son playing with wood scraps on the floor. He asked the child sweetly, "What are you making?" Just as sweetly the boy responded, "Oh, I am making a little wooden bowl for you to eat your food when you grow old." The 4-year-old smiled and went on with his work.

The words so struck the parents that they were speechless. Then tears started to stream down their cheeks. Though no words were spoken, both knew what must be done. That evening the husband took the grandfather's hand and gently led him to the family table. For the remainder of his days he ate every meal with the family. For some reason, neither the husband nor wife seemed to care any longer when a fork dropped, milk spilled, or the tablecloth soiled. — Anonymous

Delicate Fruit

This Galatians passage points out that when we yield control of our lives to the Holy Spirit, the fruit of the Spirit becomes evident.

But the fruit of the Spirit is love, joy, peace, patience, kindness, goodness, faithfulness, gentleness and self-control. — **Galatians 5:22**

These gifts are just what we need when caregiving and when sharing our thoughts and feelings. Also, take heed to the warning:

Let us not become conceited, provoking and envying each other. — **Galatians 5:26**.

Another passage that reinforces the delicate approach we should take with others is:

Do to others, as you would have them do to you.
— **Luke 6:31**

Reflection and Discussion

What does the word honor mean to you? Is it a thought or an action? What are some recent examples of how you have honored your aging loved one(s)?

What are some new ways you might honor your loved one(s)? Is God putting something heavy on your heart? Be specific with things you would like to do in the next month, three months, six months, etc.

What obstacles are you likely to face, and how might you overcome them? What is one thing you might do today or this week to honor your loved one?

What do the words obey and respect mean to you?

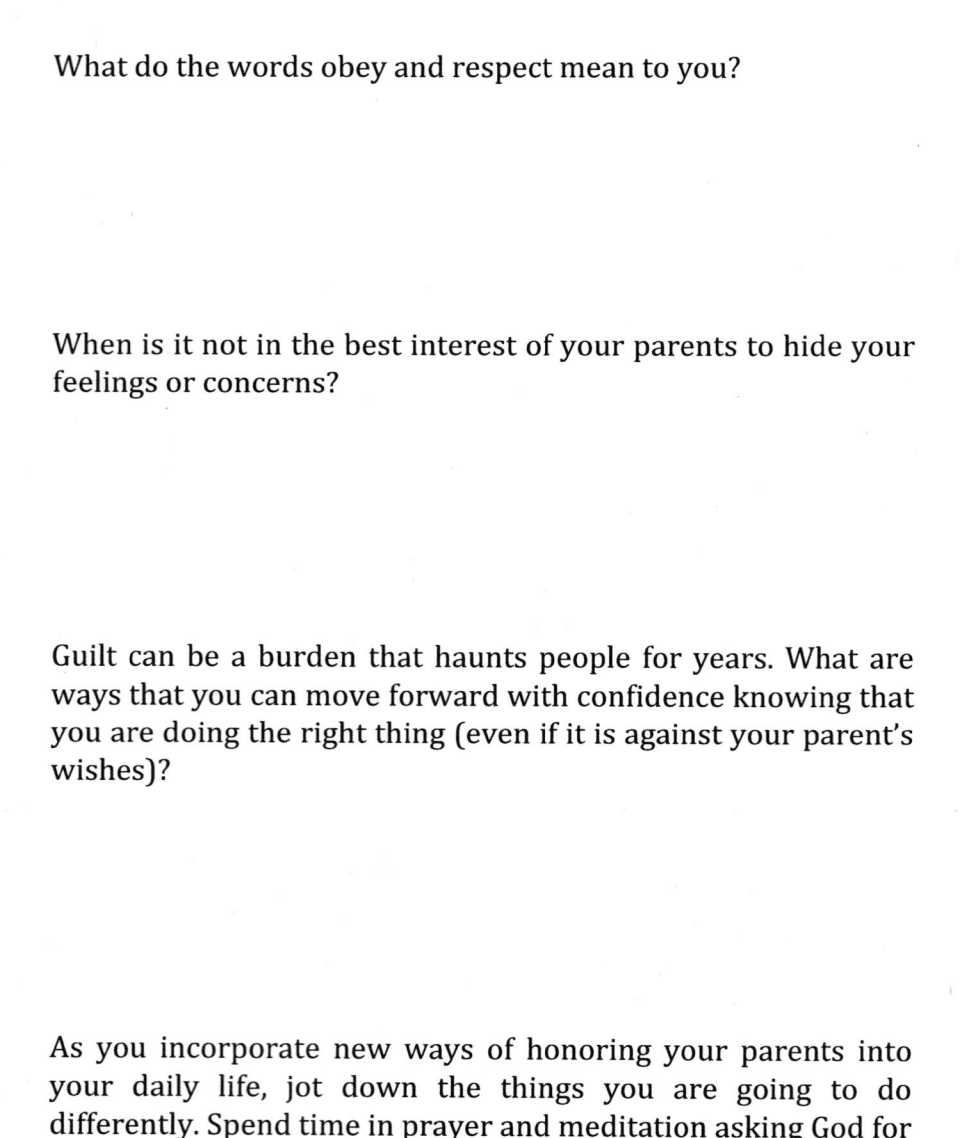

When is it not in the best interest of your parents to hide your feelings or concerns?

Guilt can be a burden that haunts people for years. What are ways that you can move forward with confidence knowing that you are doing the right thing (even if it is against your parent's wishes)?

As you incorporate new ways of honoring your parents into your daily life, jot down the things you are going to do differently. Spend time in prayer and meditation asking God for guidance, direction, healing and restoration of relationships. Then, in a month or two, look back at your list and reflect on how God has answered your prayers and how you feel about the relationship you enjoy with your parents or loved ones.

KEY LEARNINGS – *Top three findings from this chapter:*
1.
2.
3.

ACTION ITEMS - *Things you want to do or do differently:*

Check when Completed	*Action Item*	*Target Completion Date*

Prayer

Dear Heavenly Father, thank you for the precious gift of family. Thank you, Lord, for helping me to process the meaning of honor, obey and respect. I pray, Lord, that you would infuse me with Your Spirit and that You will guide my actions, words, thoughts and deeds. Help me to be aware of the struggles my loved one(s) may be facing. Help me to be compassionate and helpful in addressing the needs of others. Grant me an extra measure of strength and patience. I pray that I will honor and glorify You by the way I treat my loved one(s). In Jesus' holy and precious name. Amen.

4.
Faith in Action

In the Gospel of Luke, we find the story of two sisters who had differing styles of caring.

> *As Jesus and his disciples were on their way, he came to a village where a woman named Martha opened her home to him. She had a sister called Mary, who sat at the Lord's feet listening to what he said. But Martha was distracted by all the preparations that had to be made. She came to him and asked, "Lord, don't you care that my sister has left me to do the work by myself? Tell her to help me! Martha, Martha," the Lord answered, "you are worried and upset about many things, but only one thing is needed. Mary has chosen what is better, and it will not be take away from her."* — **Luke 10:38-42**

The story illustrates how easy it is to become task-oriented in caring for the needs of people and to forget the importance of enjoying a relationship with the ones we are serving. To a caregiver, it may seem the most urgent needs are the outward ones (*the doing*); but to a care receiver, the most important needs may be internal ones (*the being*) that can only be filled through time spent together, setting aside the chores for the moment.

It takes empathy to see the less obvious needs of our loved ones. The point of empathy is to understand, not to change or judge another's emotions and responses. To be a good helper, a person has to first understand the care receiver's needs and then be able to take appropriate action. Only when we understand can we be helpful.

The Bible shares what is expected in terms of financial and material support.

> *If anyone has material possessions and sees his brother in need but has no pity on him, how can the love of God be in him?*
> **— 1 John 3:17**

God tells us it is our responsibility to help those in need. Furthermore, as believers, our Christ-like nature should have us offering assistance.

> *Suppose you see a brother or sister who needs food or clothing, and you say, "Well, good-bye and God bless you; stay warm and eat well" — but then you don't give that person any food or clothing. What good does that do?*
> **— James 2:15-16**

Love Languages

When caring for a loved one, it is helpful to discover his or her love language. Once you determine how a person is likely to respond best, engage him or her by communicating in that love language. In his best-selling book *The Five Love Languages*, author Gary Chapman helps us understand that we all have one of the following five love languages:

1. **Words of Affirmation**

    Some people thrive on positive comments and compliments. Telling them they look good, did a great job, etc. is quite important. These people feel loved when they hear encouraging words. Without words, they may feel insecure or unimportant.

2. Quality Time

This love language is about giving your time and attention to the things someone else (e.g., your parent or spouse) values. During quality time, people are in tune with each other's inner emotions. Feelings are expressed, and there is heartfelt sharing.

3. Receiving Gifts

Some people respond best to receiving tangible symbols of love. A visible sign of love leaves the recipient feeling happy and secure in the relationship. If you are concerned about the expense, know that the money you are investing to deepen the relationship is more important than the gifts itself.

4. Acts of Service

Providing a helping hand around the house is a true expression of love to some people. It is often the simple things that show you care that mean the most. Serving another and making sacrifices requires a person to humble him or herself, especially when the chores are not glamorous.

5. Physical Touch

Lastly, some people thrive on personal touch. The response to touch can be both physical and psychological. From rubbing lotion on a person's hands or rubbing his or her back, to hugging someone or putting your arm around him or her, you will need to figure out what is soothing and comforting and what may be irritating.

Remember, just because you respond best to a particular love language does not mean your loved one will respond the same way. Much to my surprise, my wife, our three daughters and I each have a different love language.

Treasurers vs. Trust

> *After all, children should not have to save up for their parents, but parents for their children.*
> **— 2 Corinthians 12:14b**

The operative word from this 2 Corinthians passage is *should.* Should is a directional, not a definitive word. In other words, the passage does not say *do not save* for your parents. The passage states that parents *should* save for their children. Unfortunately, many older people simply have not saved enough money to retire comfortably or may have had unreasonable expectations of pension funds and Social Security benefits. So while this passage suggests that ideally it will not be necessary for children to save for their parents, many adult children will find themselves providing financial support.

While the reference in 2 Corinthians speaks of inheritance, the book of Matthew tells us that we are not to store up our treasures on earth. Matthew suggests that it is not necessary to lavish inheritance upon our children.

> *Do not store up for yourselves treasures on earth, where moth and rust destroy, and where thieves break in and steal. But store up for yourselves treasures in heaven, where moth and rust do not destroy, and where thieves do not break in and steal.* **— Matthew 6:19-20**

Providing care and covering health-related expenses can be costly, especially for people on a fixed income. So how do we know if our parents or loved ones have enough money to provide for their needs? How much is enough? To prepare for the future, one recommendation is to project care and health-related expenses with the help of a reputable and professional financial or estate planner. In Proverbs we are told of the importance of listening to advice and seeking advice.

> *Listen to advice and accept instruction, and in the end you will be wise.* — **Proverbs 19:20**

> *Make plans by seeking advice.* — **Proverbs 20:18a**

In Proverbs 19:20, the word *wise* stands out. Based on the following example from the book of Matthew, being wise would appear to be the only choice.

> *Therefore everyone who hears these words of mine and puts them into practice is like a wise man who built his house on the rock. The rain came down, the streams rose, and the winds blew and beat against that house; yet it did not fall, because it had its foundation on the rock. But everyone who hears these words of mine and does not put them into practice is like a foolish man who built his house on sand. The rain came down, the streams rose, and the winds blew and beat against that house, and it fell with a great crash.* — **Matthew 7:24-27**

In addition to professional advice, prayer is also critical. Ask God for guidance. Take time to understand the challenges you are likely to face as a loved one ages. Get an idea of the various care options and costs so that you are able to make sound and responsible decisions either with or for your aging loved one when necessary.

Who of you by worrying can add a single hour to his life?
— **Matthew 6:27**

Therefore do not worry about tomorrow, for tomorrow will worry about itself. Each day has enough trouble of its own. — **Matthew 6:34**

While the Matthew chapter 6 verses tells us not to worry about tomorrow, there is a clear difference between worrying about tomorrow and preparing for natural and expected life transitions. So, if you plan to retire at the age of 65, it is practical and consistent with biblical teachings to listen to advice, accept instruction and make plans.

While most people work to earn money to provide a certain standard of living, did you know that the Bible makes reference to retirement?

The Lord also instructed Moses, "This is the rule the Levites must follow: They must begin serving in the Tabernacle at the age of twenty-five, and they must retire at the age of fifty. After retirement they may assist their fellow Levites by serving as guards at the Tabernacle, but they may not officiate in the service. This is how you must assign duties to the Levites. — **Numbers 8:23-26 (NLT)**

If a family member faces financial difficulty, family is called to provide support.

If one of your fellow Israelites falls into poverty and is forced to sell some family land, then a close relative should buy it back for him. — **Leviticus 25:25 (NLT)**

Succession and Inheritance

The Bible refers to inheritance in two distinct ways. The first type is earthly inheritance. The second is the ultimate inheritance, the privilege of receiving God's kingdom.

Earthly inheritance is often thought of in terms of receiving assets (*e.g. money and property*) when a loved one dies. Earthly inheritance also comes in forms that are neither monetary nor tangible. While many people will not have the good fortune to receive monetary inheritance, do not overlook the inheritance that comes from good character. Maybe you have inherited a good work ethic, learned how to overcome adversity, or have an understanding of the value associated with a good reputation. The lessons we learn throughout life can be more valuable than anything tangible.

The point I like to make about receiving inheritance from family members is that it is a gift that should not be taken for granted. If you are fortunate enough to receive assets from a loved one, consider it a blessing.

There are numerous references to inheritance of assets or property in the Bible, especially in the books of Numbers and Deuteronomy. The following passage from Numbers details the order of succession when distributing an individual's personal property upon death.

> *Say to the Israelites, 'If a man dies and leaves no son, turn his inheritance over to his daughter. If he has no daughter, give his inheritance to his brothers. If he has no brothers, give his inheritance to his father's brothers. If his father had no brothers, give his inheritance to the nearest relative in his clan, that he may possess it. This is to be a legal requirement for the Israelites, as the Lord commanded Moses.'* — **Numbers 27:8-11**

In today's legal system, if a person does not make his or her wishes known prior to death through a legal document called a will, a person's assets (*not covered by a Trust or other instrument where a beneficiary is named*) will be disposed of according to an order of succession prescribed by state law.

An article from the March 2004 AARP Bulletin entitled *Will Your Ship Come In?* says family members, sons and daughters should not count on inheritance. The author of the article points out that the money people stand to inherit can come in handy regardless of the dollar amount. *"Sure, Mom and Dad will join the ranks of the dearly departed some day, but the reality is that that the day will probably come later and any inheritance is likely to be smaller than you might think. People who are 65 today can reasonably expect to live perhaps another two decades, and many intend to use that time to treat themselves to long-denied luxuries such as travel, new cars and gourmet dining. In addition, living longer means more health and long-term care costs — costs that can quickly gobble up assets."*

The safest bet is to save and plan for your own future without expecting an inheritance.

> *A good man leaves an inheritance for his children's children, but a sinner's wealth is stored up for the righteous.* — **Proverbs 13:22**

This Proverbs passage reinforces the point that sons and daughters should not count on inheritance as it suggests that people should leave their inheritance for their grandchildren, not their children.

> *Children's children are a crown to the aged, and parents are the pride of their children.* — **Proverbs 17:6**

Not only does the Bible make reference to leaving inheritance to grandchildren, in Proverbs 17:6 we learn that grandchildren are a special reward to our parents. This relationship is evident in many families where grandparents delight in and spoil grandchildren. Likewise, we see again that we should be proud of our parents.

Heavenly Rewards

While many people place value on receiving earthly possessions, the ultimate inheritance cited throughout the Bible is our relationship with the Lord while alive, and His kingdom that awaits us upon death.

They shall have no inheritance among their brothers; the Lord is their inheritance, as he promised them.
— Deuteronomy 18:2

Then the King will say to those on his right, 'Come, you who are blessed by my Father; take your inheritance, the kingdom prepared for you since the creation of the world.
— Matthew 25:34

As believers and followers of our Lord Christ Jesus, there is no better gift that we could receive than knowing that we will enjoy eternity in His presence. As the song from the group Mercy Me says, *"I can only imagine what it will be like."* Frankly, everything else pales in comparison to a life spent in heaven with the King of Kings.

Reflection and Discussion

Are you aware of your loved ones' wishes and expectations as you serve as a caregiver? On what might you want to get clarifications?

Do your parents appear to have adequate financial resources to meet their future care needs? What might your role be?

What makes it difficult for you to focus on today rather than worrying about tomorrow? What are some things you might do differently?

What expectations do you have in regards to inheritance from your parents? After giving consideration to the scriptures referenced in this section, has your opinion of the value you place on inheritance changed? Explain.

Thinking about the promise from God of the inheritance we will receive from the Lord, what might you do differently in the days ahead?

KEY LEARNINGS – *Top three findings from this chapter:*
1.
2.
3.

ACTION ITEMS - *Things you want to do or do differently:*		
Check when Completed	*Action Item*	*Target Completion Date*

Prayer

Lord, You are my rock and You never fail me. Regardless of the struggles, situations and challenges I face with my aging parent(s), I am comforted to know that You are with me. Help me to turn to You when I receive troubling news, rather than feeling anger or despair. In times of sorrow and sadness, help me to put my trust and faith in You, rather than feeling hopeless. You are a sovereign God and regardless of the circumstances I know that You will use every situation for good. Lord, comfort me and hold me in the palm of Your hand during these difficult times. Lord, guide me and direct me in all that I do. In Jesus' name. Amen.

5.
Caregiving Instruction

In 1 Timothy, God clearly indicates that taking care of our immediate family and relatives is an expectation that brings Him glory and honor.

> *But if a widow has children or grandchildren, these should learn first of all to put their religion into practice by caring for their own family and so repaying their parents and grandparents, for this is pleasing to God.* — **1 Timothy 5:4**

While this passage references widows, it points out that caring is a demonstration of our faith — *put their religion into practice by caring.* In fact, it is our responsibility to care for our own family. The word "repaying" is used to describe the adult child's responsibility to parents and grandparents and carries with it the meaning of giving back to our loved ones. In most cases, parents sacrificed, nurtured, and did for us things we could not do for ourselves. Now it is our turn to give our time, talent and treasure back to them. This is a serious commitment and duty that most are honored to fulfill.

When adults get married, the marriage vow typically says that we leave our mother and father and become one with our husband/wife. While our primary responsibility becomes our spouse and children, we do not relinquish our family ties.

When it comes to caring for family, the 1 Timothy passage clearly indicates an expectation to provide care and assistance. Caring for our family members enables us to live our faith and please God with all that we do.

In another 1 Timothy passage, God clearly indicates how He feels about those who neglect their families.

> *If anyone does not provide for his relatives, and especially for his immediate family, he has denied the faith and is worse than an unbeliever.*
> **— 1 Timothy 5:8**

An operative word in this passage is "provide." Webster's defines this as *"To furnish; supply: provide food and shelter for a family; to make available; to set down as a stipulation; and to make ready ahead of time; prepare."* The word "provide" is a verb indicating action is involved. The second part of the passage clearly states that if we do not uphold our responsibility, we are not being faithful to God and are worse than an unbeliever.

It strikes me that by knowing our responsibility and failing to do what is expected of us is worse than, not equivalent to, a nonbeliever. A nonbeliever simply does not know better, but believers are expected to know better and to provide care for our families. Giving back, providing care and support, and demonstrating our love in all that we do is pleasing to God and is expected.

No Dispensation for Distance

Our responsibility to honor our parents is regardless of our geographic location and how many miles separate us from our loved ones. We also have the responsibility to look out for our friends and neighbors.

Never abandon a friend — either yours or your father's. Then in your time of need, you won't have to ask your relatives for assistance. It is better to go to a neighbor than to a relative who lives far away.
— **Proverbs 27:10-12** (NLT)

The Proverbs passage emphasizes our responsibility to come to the aid of others. Caring for one another is more than just tending to the needs of our immediate family. Rather, we are called to provide care and support to our community of friends and neighbors.

This is not to suggest that adult children should shrug their responsibility to provide care and support for parents who live out of town. Instead, in situations where family lives out of town, others can and should supplement the care provided by family members.

People often compare young, dependent children to older adults requiring care. As loved ones face functional challenges due to aging or illness, they may become dependent on family and friends for help with daily living activities. These activities are fundamental to caring for one's self and maintaining independence. If you live in a distant city or are otherwise unable to provide assistance, do not overlook or minimize your loved ones' needs.

The two types of activities of daily living are personal care and independent living. While both are critically important, people tend to focus on one or the other.

- Activities of daily living (ADLs) are everyday personal care activities such as bathing, dressing, getting in or out of bed or a chair (also called transferring), using the toilet, eating, and getting around or walking.

- Instrumental activities of daily living (IADLs) are activities related to independent living and include preparing meals, managing money (writing checks, paying bills), shopping for groceries or personal items, maintaining a residence/performing housework (e.g., laundry, cleaning), taking medications, using a telephone, handling mail, and traveling via car or public transportation.

In addition to daily living activities, which tend to be task-oriented, don't overlook the need for spiritual and emotional support. Caring for one another is all about enhancing the quality of life, maximizing dignity, providing encouragement, and helping make the lives of loved ones easier and more enjoyable.

Carrying The Burden

Carry each other's burdens, and in this way you will fulfill the law of Christ. — **Galatians 6:2**

The Galatians passage references carrying each other's burdens, and indicates that by doing so, we fulfill the law of Christ. I am often reminded of how the needs of our children dictate the things we will do over the course of the day. For example, our children need to be driven to and from school at specific times. If they participate in extracurricular activities and sports, we are responsible for getting them to and from activities and to enthusiastically support them at recitals, school plays and games. I believe this is a logical application of Galatians 6:2.

Just as it may not be someone's first choice to watch a soccer game in the rain on a chilly Saturday morning, or to attend out of town competitions weekend after weekend, we do it with joy and as a demonstration of our love and support. Just as we meet our children's needs according to the schedule that is set for us, we should make time to address the needs the needs of our loved ones' who are aging or ill.

If your child is sick and needs to see a doctor, what parent would not miss a day of work to see that he or she receives the proper medical attention? Are you ready and willing to do the same for your parent? As we consider our responsibilities to care for our parents, we face a number of choices.

Know that you are not alone, and you do not need to do everything on your own. Fortunately, there are many wonderful organizations and programs that can supplement what you are able to do and provide the level and type of care deemed appropriate for your situation. Services are available to help with everything from providing functional assessments to home-delivered meals and companion care provided in the comfort of a person's own home. Just as God enables us to rise to each new occasion or challenge, trust that He will equips you with the resources you need at the appropriate time.

Expressing Yourself

When faced with a stressful situation, people generally do not communicate their thoughts well. Later, people may have regrets about things they either said or did not say. When expressing yourself to family members, be careful to:

Say What You Mean,
Mean What You Say.
Just Don't Say It Mean!

Pleasant words are sweet to the soul — they are heartfelt. A cheerful heart helps us to smile brighter, hug tighter, and live lighter *(free from the bondage of our sin.)*

Pleasant words are a honeycomb, sweet to the soul and healing to the bones. — **Proverbs 16:24**

In fact, pleasant words are healing to our bones. Bones are an infrastructure. If one part of the infrastructure is fragile, frail or flawed, the whole body is a risk and may fail.

A cheerful heart is good medicine, but a crushed spirit dries up the bones. — **Proverbs 17:22**

Pleasant words are also said to be good medicine. While it can be so easy to find fault in any situation, the real challenge can be looking for the good in everything. God is a perfect example. He knows we are sinners down to the very core of our being, yet, He loves us and lifts us up. The choice is ours. We can take the negative or the "*My glass is half empty*" approach. Or, we can share kind words, look for the good in everything, and live a life better represented by the "*My glass is half full*" attitude.

Variety – The Spice of Life

Birth order and many other things contribute to personalities, styles and the things we say and do. While some people think the world would be a much better place if everyone did as they chose, the fact is that we are all different by God's design.

Teach me, and I will be quiet; show me where I have been wrong. How painful are honest words! But what do your arguments prove? — **Job 6:24-25**

In the Job passage, the first two words are teach me, not *lose patience with me, scream at me and leave the room in a huff*, or *give up on me*. If we believe someone is wrong, notice it does not say *rub salt on the wound*, or *have a chip on your shoulder for being so smart.* As the scripture indicates, arguments do not prove anything. In many cases, arguments show our immaturity and our inability to cope with life issues.

Notice that the Job passage says *how painful are honest words*, not *avoid honest words because they can be painful*. Family dynamics can be quite challenging. Do not put off the tough discussions for another day; instead, talk in a manner that is consistent with the Golden Rule.

We all see things differently, and talking to someone with a different perspective and personality may help us understand things we would not otherwise recognize. Many times, we find that once families are able to express themselves truthfully, clearly and appropriately, they can begin to work toward a solution, often more quickly than expected.

> *Starting a quarrel is like breaching a dam; so drop the matter before a dispute breaks out.*
> **— Proverbs 17:14**

It can be hurtful to be shown you are wrong. Some people choose to defend a position they know is wrong, rather than give in and admit they made a mistake.

The Proverbs passage uses the word quarrel, suggesting something is trivial as if two people are looking for something about which to bicker. The advice given is to drop the matter before a dispute breaks out.

With more substantive challenges that may cause a breakdown in the relationship, avoiding the issues or stuffing your feelings may not be best. Consider your motivation and purpose of anything you might say. If you think what you are about to say is going to cause problems, consider if it is worth the conflict.

We have all heard the saying *"You can't see the forest through the trees."* People are often so close to the problem that they do not see the bigger picture and what may be an obvious solution to a problem.

If your family is struggling with conflict and disagreement, make sure to spend time in prayer before engaging in any discussion. Ask the Lord to help everyone deal with the issues at hand in fairness and truth. Pray that the more outspoken members of the family will take their turn listening, and pray that the Lord with help the quieter one's have the courage to speak up and share their thoughts. More than anything, pray that the Lord will help everyone involved realize the ultimate goal is not who wins and loses; rather, what is best and necessary for your loved ones for whom everyone is concerned. Lay your burdens at the foot of the cross and ask God to open minds and soften hearts, as He impresses upon everyone His wishes and will.

What Did You Mean by That?

People often use everyday words to describe or explain something; however, family members might interpret the words differently. For example, close your eyes and think of the color blue. Now ask others in your family to describe in detail the color blue about which they were thinking. If you are like most families, the blues were not the same. If there is disagreement about an issue related to aging, illness or care, do not simply assume that others are out to get you. It could be a simple misunderstanding or a difference in communication styles.

Families are often faced with making difficult decisions on short notice. In these situations, stress can be tremendous. Now, introduce family dynamics and brace yourself. These are times when families need to unite for the benefit and well-being of loved ones. Do not let the situation tear your family apart or burden loved ones with arguments.

Are you the one in the family who is outspoken? Maybe it's time to give someone else a chance to talk. Are you the one who tends to be more reserved or withdrawn? Plan your words carefully. While your words might be few, they can still be powerful.

Remember, people do not read each other's minds. Therefore, if you do not express yourself, do not expect anyone else to know what you are thinking.

> *"Instead, speaking the truth in love, we will in all things grow up into him who is the Head, that is, Christ."*
> — **Ephesians 4:15**

As the Ephesians passage says, *speak the truth in love*. The truth can set you free. Remain calm, share and explain what you are thinking and suggesting and give reasons why. Talk and give each other turns to paraphrase and ask questions as necessary. Do not exaggerate and try to avoid becoming overly emotional.

> *My dear brothers, take note of this: Everyone should be quick to listen, slow to speak and slow to become angry.*
> — **James 1:19**

When discussing issues that may be controversial or invoke emotion, try asking questions instead of making opinionated statements. The reasons being:

- Opinionated statements have a tendency to come across as negative and undermining if people have different opinions. For example, if you say something like, "*It makes no sense to me why ...,*" the person to whom that is directed is likely to become defensive.

- On the other hand, questions have a tendency to suggest a desire to understand, an openness to discuss and a willingness to work together. For example, "*What is your thought on ... ? Do you think there might be another way to ... ?*"

The Job 6:24-25 passage, referenced as few pages earlier, also uses the word *quiet.* God gave us each two ears and one mouth. Are you listening twice as much as you are speaking? When talking, it can be very difficult to hear and learn. The more a conversation is dominated by one or two people, the further entrenched in their position and beliefs they tend to become. At the same time, other family members tend to build up resentment. Much of this can be avoided by giving everyone a chance to talk and be heard.

Set Reasonable Expectations

It may be best to start by reaching a common understanding of the situation during an initial family discussion, rather than trying to reach a decision. Remember, you cannot change anyone else but yourself. Andy Rooney of *60 Minutes* offered some great advice:

I've Learned...
- That being kind is more important than being right.
- That I can always pray for someone when I don't have the strength to help him in some other way.
- That sometimes all a person needs is a hand to hold and a heart to understand.
- That under everyone's hard shell is someone who wants to be appreciated and loved.
- That the Lord didn't do it all in one day. What makes me think I can?

- That to ignore the facts does not change the facts.
- That I can't choose how I feel, but I can choose what I do about it.

A Helping Hand

Caregivers often become exhausted and burnt out caring for their loved ones while trying to handle all their other responsibilities — family, work, church, community, etc. Caregiving can be quite demanding, and I encourage you to seek and to accept support from others.

When people ask how they can be supportive, most are serious about their desire to help. The problem is that when someone makes a comment like, *"Let me know how I can help,"* the burden of following up is on the caregiver or the care receiver. Chances are, you don't want to be a burden to your family and friends.

When people ask how they can help, be prepared to respond with a specific request. If nothing comes to mind at that moment, write down their names and get back to them. If you yourself are not sure what type of support may be most helpful, consider this: Care receivers tend to need three types of support:

- Emotional support is more about being than doing. It is relational.

- Informational support has to do with becoming aware and gaining knowledge that may be helpful now or in the future. It can also involve skill-building and helping others process information and make informed decisions.

- Instrumental support involves hands-on assistance with daily living activities. While a person might be functionally able to do things on his or her own, don't underestimate the value of a helping hand. Things others can do to make life easier tend to be much appreciated.

The book of Exodus (18:13-23) shares the story of Moses caring for the Israelites. When Moses was leading God's people from Egypt to their homeland, he was overwhelmed with his responsibility. Jethro expressed concern that Moses was going to wear himself out and that he could not handle the burden all by himself. Fortunately Moses accepted the life-changing advice from his father-in-law and found others to help carry the load. As caregivers, we too need to recognize our limitations, delegate tasks and accept the help and advice of people we trust.

> *The next day Moses took his seat to serve as judge for the people, and they stood around him from morning till evening. When his father-in-law saw all that Moses was doing for the people, he said, "What is this you are doing for the people? Why do you alone sit as judge, while all these people stand around you from morning till evening?" Moses answered him, "Because the people come to me to seek God's will. Whenever they have a dispute, it is brought to me, and I decide between the parties and inform them of God's decrees and laws." Moses' father-in-law replied, "What you are doing is not good. You and these people who come to you will only wear yourselves out. The work is too heavy for you; you cannot handle it alone. Listen now to me and I will give you some advice, and may God be with you. You must be the people's representative before God and bring their disputes to him. Teach them the decrees and laws, and show them the way to live and the duties they are to perform. But*

select capable men from all the people — men who fear God, trustworthy men who hate dishonest gain — and appoint them as officials over thousands, hundreds, fifties and tens. Have them serve as judges for the people at all times, but have them bring every difficult case to you; the simple cases they can decide themselves. That will make your load lighter, because they will share it with you. If you do this and God so commands, you will be able to stand the strain, and all these people will go home satisfied."

— **Exodus 18:13-23**

Reflection and Discussion

What do the words care and provide mean to you? What are specific examples of how you might provide care for your aging loved one in a manner that would be pleasing to God?

What are some of the things that tend to divert you from your responsibility to your family? How might you handle or prioritize things differently so you can care for your parent?

What are some sacrifices you need to make in your daily life to honor God, yourself and your parents? How might making sacrifices send a clear message to your children of what is important and what is expected?

While making sacrifices is not easy, these are instructions from God. Know that God will give you the strength and the wisdom to help you carry out His will. Spend time in prayer asking God for direction and encouragement so that you can fulfill your family responsibilities.

Caregiving Instruction

KEY LEARNINGS – *Top three findings from this chapter:*
1.
2.
3.

ACTION ITEMS - *Things you want to do or do differently:*

Check when Completed	*Action Item*	*Target Completion Date*

Prayer

Dear Lord of heaven and earth, when circumstances cause me to feel overwhelmed, help me to remember that You are my refuge. I trust in You and know that You use all situations for good. Your Word and Your promises give me strength. May Your Holy Spirit fill my heart and guide me one day at a time. I love You with all of my heart, and I thank You for Your unwavering love. In Jesus' name. Amen.

6.
Love and Support

Three of the most powerful words in the English language are the words *"I LOVE YOU."*

When I think of love, I think of how I love my wife and children. I think of sharing in their joy and their pain. I think of my role as a father in terms of encourager, defender, teacher and coach.

The attributes of love are spelled out in the book of 1 Corinthians (13:4-8).

- *Love* is patient
- *Love* is kind
- *Love* does not envy
- *Love* is not proud
- *Love* is not rude
- *Love* is not self-seeking
- *Love* is not easily angered
- *Love* keeps no record of wrongs
- *Love* does not delight in evil but rejoices with the truth
- *Love* always protects, always trusts, always hopes, and always perseveres
- *Love* never fails

A wonderful demonstration of love is the story of Jacob in the book of Genesis. In this story, Jacob was in love with Rachel, Laban's youngest daughter. Jacob agreed to work for Laban for seven years in exchange for his daughter's hand in marriage.

> *So Jacob served seven years to get Rachel, but they seemed like only a few days to him because of his love for her.* — **Genesis 29:20**

Imagine loving someone so much that you give of yourself for years and years, and it only seems like a few days. While the story of Jacob is about love that leads to marriage, the story of caregiving is about love and honor that leads to dignity and quality of life. Both are powerful expressions of love.

It strikes me that the difference between the words *live* and *love* is one letter — i. The reason I mention these two words is because the Bible is a love letter from God. In His love letter, He teaches us how we can live an abundant life — a life of love, joy, freedom and peace. So often the thing that holds us back from loving and living is the 'I' — the person who stares back at you when you look at yourself in the mirror. It is our sins, our selfishness, our busyness, our coveting and more that keeps us from living the abundant life.

The other letter difference between the words live and love is o. The symbols that come to mind are Xs and Os representing hugs and kisses. Think of our Father, Abba, and His desire to hold us in His arms to comfort us, protect us and remind us of His unfailing love. Think of Him modeling a relationship for us and with us. So here's the question; how do you think of love when you think of your parents? How can you love more and live freer? What is holding you back?

Did you know that there are three different kinds of love? They are Eros (*physical*), Philia (*interpersonal or relationship*), and Agape (*divine and unconditional*). Love is a gift from God, and the more we love God, the more likely we are to love others.

> *Jesus replied, "The most important commandment is this: 'Listen, O Israel! The Lord our God is the one and only Lord. And you must love the Lord your God with all your heart, all your soul, all your mind, and all your strength.' The second is equally important: 'Love your neighbor as yourself.' No other commandment is greater than these."*
> — **Mark 12:29-31 (NLT)**

Notice how the Mark passage uses the singular word *commandment* and then refers to the plural *these*. That's because the love of God and the love of people go together. In the book of 1 John, the connection is made between loving God and keeping his commandments, such as loving our neighbors and honoring our parents.

> *If someone claims, "I know God," but doesn't obey God's commandments, that person is a liar and is not living in the truth. But those who obey God's word truly show how completely they love him. That is how we know we are living in him.* — **1 John 2:4-5 (NLT)**

Don't Take Love For Granted

When you visit with loved ones, do you tell them, "*I love you*?" I often observe people who say things in a round-about way. The words *I love you* are often diluted and said more as a salutation. For example, instead of saying goodbye, many people substitute the words *I love you*. If you have not recently shared an honest to goodness heartfelt *I love you*, try holding someone's hands, looking him or her straight in the eyes and deliberately saying, "*I love you.*"

In addition to the words *I love you*, consider expressing your feelings and keeping in touch with tangible expressions of love such as cards and flowers, visits, e-mails and telephone calls. It is always nice to know that someone is thinking of you and that they care. One of the greatest needs of the human heart is the need for significance. People want to know their lives are important and have meaning. They want to know they are loved and accepted even when they may act and feel unacceptable. A simple expression of love goes a long way.

Most of the people I talk with say that after a loved one dies, they wish they would have said I love you more often. Also, people often question if a loved one really knew in his or her heart how much they were loved and appreciated. My point is, do not assume or take love for granted. Say it! Mean it! Show it!

> *Dear children, let us not love with words or tongue but with actions and in truth.* — **1 John 3:18**

Forgiveness and Reconciliation

While the words *I love you* are a few of the most powerful words, the words *I'm sorry* can be some of the most difficult to say. When we experience conflict, many people would rather forget than forgive. However, forgetting rarely works. Things said or done that have been hurtful for someone can be embedded in the heart.

> *And when you stand praying, if you hold anything against anyone, forgive him, so that your Father in heaven may forgive you your sins.* — **Mark 11:25**

Each and every day we sin. However, Jesus is our model for forgiveness. Think of the song Amazing Grace and how God "saved a wretch like me". We are all sinners. Regardless of whether our sins are sins of omission or commission, what is totally awesome is that God sent his Son, Jesus Christ, to pay the ultimate price. Through His grace and mercy, He forgives us of all our sins — past, present and future.

> *In him we have redemption through his blood, the forgiveness of sins, in accordance with the riches of God's grace.* — **Ephesians 1:7**

In fact, when God forgives, He wipes the slate clean. A clean slate is important not only for your parents' offenses, but also yours. You might find it easy to focus on things you wish you had done differently in your relationship with your parents. Do not fall into the trap of limiting the quality relationship you can have with them now by feeling guilty about the past. Do not dwell on regret. Recognize what you could have done differently. If appropriate, ask for your parents' and God's forgiveness and then move on to making this time with them as special as possible.

When you have conflict with someone, do you forgive the other person and wipe the slate clean (*regardless of whether there has been an apology or not*)? Chances are, we forgive, but never really forget. Both are needed and necessary, and are two different and distinct steps. When we truly forgive, we treat others as if something that was offensive to us never took place. Forgetting can be difficult; however, it is the Christ-like thing to do. It is important when a similar situation occurs in the future not to react based on memories, but to act based on biblical principles. If you are struggling to forgive someone, how can you expect God to forgive you? As the Lord's Prayer says:

> *... and forgive us our sins, just as we have forgiven those who have sinned against us.* — **Matthew 6:12 (NLT)**

The most common Greek word in the New Testament for forgiveness carries the meaning of being pardoned or released from the penalty of our sins. God forgives us of our sins when we repent (*regret our sins and turn from them*) and believe that Jesus Christ suffered and died in our place to pay the penalty of our sin. When we become a follower of Christ, we are justified (*God chooses to see us as perfectly acceptable as though we had never sinned*), reconciled to God, and given new life.

But God demonstrates his own love for us in this: While we were still sinners, Christ died for us. Since we have now been justified by his blood, how much more shall we be saved from God's wrath through him! For if, when we were God's enemies, we were reconciled to him through the death of his Son, how much more, having been reconciled, shall we be saved through his life! Not only is this so, but we also rejoice in God through our Lord Jesus Christ, through whom we have now received reconciliation. — **Romans 5:8-11.**

It is also important to distinguish how forgiveness and making amends are different. Forgiveness is the act of forgiving when a person has harmed you. Making amends has to do with making things right when you have harmed someone.

Looking Ahead

Every day, families unexpectedly face health-related crisis situations. It is often at these times that we realize that we should have done more to prepare but did not. When in crisis, the failure to anticipate and understand long-term care needs and discuss the consequences, creates family-wide implications affecting physical, emotional and spiritual health. Regardless of how well a person planned for their retirement years, even the best laid plans can crumble.

Come to me, all you who are weary and burdened, and I will give you rest. — **Matthew 11:28**

If you spend your time looking in the rearview mirror to see what is behind you, it is just a matter of time before you crash. Instead of looking back, focus on:

"Forgetting what is behind and straining toward what is ahead." — **Philippians 3:13b**

Put the circumstances of your past behind you and get on with the wonderful plan God has in store for you. God wants us to live for today.

Therefore, do not worry about tomorrow, for tomorrow will worry about itself. Each day has enough trouble of its own. — **Matthew 6:34**

We all have certain regrets. Thankfully, God forgives us. Maybe it is time for you to truly forgive yourself. Stop beating yourself up for bad choices of the past, repent and move forward.

Being Kind

Be kind and compassionate to one another, forgiving each other, just as in Christ God forgave you.
— **Ephesians 4:32**

Sometimes, we are so wrapped up in our own lives that we simply tune out others. The Ephesians passage tells us to be both kind and compassionate. I'm not sure that either can stand alone. Being kind reflects how we act, react and treat others. Being compassionate reflects the sincerity of our heart and our genuine concern. Are you putting the needs of others before yourself? Are you best described as selfish or selfless?

Do nothing out of selfish ambition or vain conceit, but in humility consider others better than yourselves. Each of you should look not only to your own interests, but also to the interests of others. Your attitude should be the same as that of Christ Jesus: — **Philippians 2:3-5**

If family dynamics have been a challenge in the past, let kindness prevail from this day forward and take whatever steps are necessary to mend family relationships. Also, as you express your feelings, watch the tone of your voice and instead of using the word *you*, think of how you can use the word *I*. Instead of placing blame, take ownership for your own feelings and actions. For example, instead of saying, "*You hurt me years ago when …* ," change your words around. Instead, say, "*I have felt hurt since our disagreement years ago and have a hard time understanding why …* "

Actions vs. Reactions

Personal responsibility is the common element of the following passages:

Above all, love each other deeply, because love covers over a multitude of sins. — **1 Peter 4:8**

Anyone who hates his brother is a murderer, and you know that no murderer has eternal life in him.
— **1 John 3:15**

In 1 Peter we are told that *Above all,* we must *love each other deeply*. Why? Because love covers a multitude of sins. In 1 John, we are told that if we hate our brother, we are living against God's word.

In Psalms 34:14, we are told *Turn from evil and do good; seek peace and pursue it.* Notice how it does not say *tell your sibling or relative to turn from evil.* Rather it implies that the responsibility is on us. We are also told to be peacemakers in Matthew 5: *"Seek peace and pursue it."* All of these passages refer to our personal responsibility regardless of the past.

What happens if you attempt to make amends and forgive others and they do not respond? If you have tried in a Christ-like manner to mend the relationship, do not worry about the other person's reaction. At the same time, do not rationalize your efforts believing that you have done all that you can, when your attempt may not have been whole-hearted.

"If it is possible, as far as it depends on you, live at peace with everyone." — **Romans 12:18.**

Focus on doing what is right. Also, just as God's grace and mercy is not a one-time thing, your actions and words should be consistent over time and not simply a one-time effort. Let your life reflect the loving, kind and caring character that God shows us each and every day.

A strategy that works well for me when I get upset with someone is to sit down at my computer and simply write a letter. While I don't send the letter to the person who has frustrated me, I simply want to get all the negative stuff out of my mind and body and onto paper. Then once I am finished, I read it, shred it and go on with my life. The point is do not try to cover it up — get it out.

Advice and Counsel

Just as Jesus closely surrounded himself with 12 disciples, there are numerous passages that demonstrate the importance of friends and seeking guidance. Three common sources of guidance and strength for caregivers are community assistance, friends and God and His promises to us. Caregivers have unique circumstances that affect the resources available to them. Some may live where community assistance is limited, some may have a small circle of friends and family, and some may not understand how God supplies joy and strength for our service as caregivers. Ask God for His help and provision with your needs before you exhaust yourself with your own efforts.

If any of you lacks wisdom, he should ask God, who gives generously to all without finding fault, and it will be given to him. But when he asks, he must believe and not doubt, because he who doubts is like a wave of the sea, blown and tossed by the wind. That man should not think he will receive anything from the Lord; — **James 1:5-7**

Caregiving decisions are not to be made lightly, but decisions will have to be made. God is never annoyed when we come to Him in faith and ask for wisdom. He will provide.

The way of a fool seems right to him, but a wise man listens to advice. — **Proverbs 12:15**

In the Proverbs passage we are told that we do not and will not ever know any better unless we seek the advice of others. When I think of seeking advice, I think of people who have greater knowledge and wisdom than me. This suggests seeking others who have already faced similar challenges associated with aging and caregiving. Let them share their wisdom and experiences for your good. We need to make each precious day count.

Teach us to number our days alright, that we may gain a heart of wisdom. — **Psalm 90:12**

Twice the Blessings, Half the Burden

> *Two are better than one, because they have a good return for their work: If one falls down, his friend can help him up. But pity the man who falls and has no one to help him up!* — **Ecclesiastes 4:9-10**

I believe that not only are two minds better than one, but additionally, with two people we receive twice the blessing and carry only half the burden. We are not meant to live life alone and rely solely on ourselves.

> *Again, I tell you that if two of you on earth agree about anything you ask for, it will be done for you by my Father in heaven. For where two or three come together in my name, there am I with them.* — **Matthew 18:19-20**

I love how the passage from Matthew begins: *Again, I tell you...* The word again suggests that we did not hear or understand the importance of this the first time. Also, His promise is not guaranteed if we are alone facing struggles, only if we are standing with at least one other person. The power of friendship with our brothers and sisters in Christ is amazing!

The concept in Ecclesiastes is two are better than one. We learn the importance of having a support network. Chances are, somewhere along your journey as a caregiver, you are going to fall down. The Bible suggests pity, as if you should have known better than to not have a support network, friend or mentor that can help you through difficult times.

God often reveals himself to us through our friends. He sends friends to us as much for comfort as for advice. Think of the following passages:

> *A friend loves at all times, and a brother is born for adversity.* — **Proverbs 17:17**

I command you to love each other in the same way that I love you. And here is how to measure it — the greatest love is shown when people lay down their lives for their friends. — **John 15:12-13 (NLT)**

Basically, a friend in need is a friend in deed. We need friends to survive and thrive in life. I recently saw a video that demonstrates the importance of friends. The video had to do with a piece of charcoal. The rather profound example indicated that when a lit piece of charcoal is separated from others, it will soon extinguish itself. However, once placed back with the others, it soon starts burning again. In the same way, we all need friends to keep us going. The encouragement of friends can be critical, especially as new caregiving challenges unexpectedly emerge.

Reflection and Discussion

How does the definition of love in the Corinthians passage relate to your relationship with your loved one who is aging or ill? What are some ways that you can express your love for your parents, other family members or friends?

When was the last time you told your parent(s) that you love them? Who might you want to share some honest words with in your family?

What would be a likely response if you opened a family discussion with prayer? What would be some of the things you might pray for?

What are things that make a conversation difficult? How might you approach the conversation? What are some areas or issues where you have a strong opinion that could ultimately cause conflict and arguing? What might you do to avoid quarrels?

What events from your past are you finding challenging to release? With whom might you want to make amends?

KEY LEARNINGS – *Top three findings from this chapter:*

1.

2.

3.

ACTION ITEMS - *Things you want to do or do differently:*

Check when Completed	Action Item	Target Completion Date

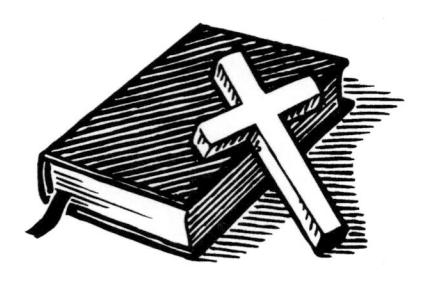

Prayer

Lord God, help me to become more like You in my relationships with my family members. During these difficult times, help me to remember that everyone is trying to help and do what is best. Lord, I pray that You will fill me with an extra measure of your Spirit to guide me. When I am in disagreement with someone, help me not to respond in anger, selfishness, arrogance or pride, but in humility, understanding that it is Your will that will prevail. Help me Lord to have a servant's attitude and be loving and kind in all that I do. Lord, I pray that through our differences, we come together as a family in our faith and our love. In Jesus' name. Amen.

7.
Peace and Purpose

Death is a fact of life everyone must deal with at one time or another. Death helps show us what living really is all about. Death should not be a topic that families avoid talking about. While the following scripture refers to being willing to die for our faith, it shares important principles about death that I believe merit consideration.

> *Yes, we live under constant danger of death because we serve Jesus, so that the life of Jesus will be evident in our dying bodies. So we live in the face of death, but this has resulted in eternal life for you. But we continue to preach because we have the same kind of faith the psalmist had when he said, "I believed in God, so I spoke." We know that God, who raised the Lord Jesus, will also raise us with Jesus and present us to himself together with you. All of this is for your benefit. And as God's grace reaches more and more people, there will be great thanksgiving, and God will receive more and more glory. That is why we never give up. Though our bodies are dying, our spirits are being renewed every day. For our present troubles are small and won't last very long. Yet they produce for us a glory that vastly outweighs them and will last forever! So we don't look at the troubles we can see now; rather, we fix our gaze on things that cannot be seen. For the*

things we see now will soon be gone, but the things we cannot see will last forever.
— **2 Corinthians 4:11-20**

Give Proper Consideration

As believers, we should be comforted to know we are going to a much better place. Once God says our work here is finished and calls us home, we will rejoice in the fact that for eternity we will be with our Lord. The verses from Ecclesiastes make it clear that we should be giving consideration to issues directly related to death.

It is better to spend your time at funerals than at festivals. For you are going to die, and you should think about it while there is still time. Sorrow is better than laughter, for sadness has a refining influence on us. A wise person thinks much about death, while the fool thinks only about having a good time now. — **Ecclesiastes 7:2-4 (NLT)**

Again the Bible references the word wise, and we are told that it is wise to think about death. We are even told that if all we do is think about having a good time now, we are foolish. Often people avoid things that are difficult rather than facing them head on. Unfortunately, many people think about having a good time now simply because they don't know what to do, whom to call, or how to help.

People who have never experienced the death of a loved one are often challenged to prepare for or anticipate death, let alone deal with the uncertainty and mystery associated with death. Talking about death can uncover struggles a person may be having.

Since the children have flesh and blood, he too shared in their humanity so that by his death he might destroy him who holds the power of death — that is, the devil — and free those who all their lives were held in slavery by their fear of death. — **Hebrews 2:14-15**

Aging and death can be unsettling for those who live only for this life. But even those who believe in Christ can feel anxious when they think of moving from the known to the unknown. Jesus understood this human anxiety so He prepared His disciples for His own death with the following words:

Do not let your hearts be troubled. Trust in God; trust also in me. In my Father's house are many rooms; if it were not so, I would have told you. I am going there to prepare a place for you. And if I go and prepare a place for you, I will come back and take you to be with me that you also may be where I am. You know the way to the place where I am going." — **John 14:1-4**

For Christians, death is not the end of life; it is the beginning of an eternal adventure of indescribable wonder and joy. When we live our lives with our hearts in communion with Jesus, we are never quite at home here. Paul the Apostle understood this when he wrote this:

For to me, to live is Christ and to die is gain. If I am to go on living in the body, this will mean fruitful labor for me. Yet what shall I choose? I do not know! I am torn between the two: I desire to depart and be with Christ, which is better by far. — **Philippians 1:21-23**

The good news is that nothing can separate us from the love of Christ. After all, being with Christ in heaven is the ultimate prize for those who believe.

Who shall separate us from the love of Christ? Shall trouble or hardship or persecution or famine or nakedness or danger or sword? As it is written: "For your sake we face death all day long; we are considered as sheep to be slaughtered." No, in all these things we are more than conquerors through him who loved us. For I am convinced that neither death nor life, neither angels nor demons, neither the present nor the future, nor any powers, neither height nor depth, nor anything else in all creation, will be able to separate us from the love of God that is in Christ Jesus our Lord. — **Romans 8:35-39**

While death is inevitable for all of us, I believe it is important for family members to share their wishes. We can only honor a loved one's final wishes if we know what they are. Here's an example of a parent sharing his final wishes with his son:

Joseph threw himself upon his father and wept over him and kissed him. Then Joseph directed the physicians in his service to embalm his father Israel. So the physicians embalmed him, taking a full forty days, for that was the time required for embalming. And the Egyptians mourned for him seventy days. When the days of mourning had passed, Joseph said to Pharaoh's court, "If I have found favor in your eyes, speak to Pharaoh for me. Tell him, 'My father made me swear an oath and said, "I am about to die; bury me in the tomb I dug for myself in the land of Canaan." Now let me go up and bury my father; then I will return.'" Pharaoh said, "Go up and bury your father, as he made you swear to do." — **Genesis 50:1-6**

Living Legacy

Jesus left us the ultimate legacy — His Word. As we spend time in His Word, we are reminded of His character, His teachings and our purpose.

And I will make every effort to see that after my departure you will always be able to remember these things.
— **2 Peter 1:15**

Jesus left His legacy. How will you and your loved ones be remembered? Just as Jesus planned for His departure, give some consideration to legacies within your family. What are you and your parents going to leave behind for the benefit of others? If you are uncertain about your legacy, there's no time like the present to begin creating one that you would be happy to have live on long after you are gone.

A great way to plan ahead is to write your own obituary and epitaph. What are the focal points?

- Your success or your significance?
- Your personality or your purpose?

Planning ahead can be a wonderful learning experience and a time to share in fond memories. We should truly capitalize on this time spent together so that we have more than just a few pictures and select memories which, over time, fade away.

Final Arrangements

Eventually, all of us must decide how we would prefer others to dispose of our remains. As we consider our arrangements, it is important to remember that God cares more about our eternal souls than our temporary housing. Making a decision for cremation or burial is not a biblical decision; rather it is a personal preference. For some, this decision may be based on upbringing or our affiliation with a church or denomination. For others it may be based on cost. A burial tends to be more expensive as there are a number of additional expenses that are not associated with cremation.

The following passages reference both the burial and cremation of the dead.

You, however, will go to your fathers in peace and be buried at a good old age. — **Genesis 15:15**

After burying him, he said to his sons, "When I die, bury me in the grave where the man of God is buried; lay my bones beside his bones. — ***1 Kings 13:31***

...all their valiant men journeyed through the night to Beth Shan. They took down the bodies of Saul and his sons from the wall of Beth Shan and went to Jabesh, where they burned them. — **1 Samuel 31:12**

You turn men back to dust, saying, "Return to dust, O sons of men. — **Psalm 90:3**

All go to the same place; all come from dust, and to dust all return. — **Ecclesiastes 3:20**

While making the decision on how to handle a body upon death can be difficult for many, when God calls us home, the real question is not about our physical remains, but about our souls.

The Grieving Process

Grieving is a process of acknowledging, accepting and working through loss. While often associated with death, grieving also occurs when there is loss resulting from illness or disease at the final stage of life. For example, Alzheimer's causes a cognitive or mental loss. Cancer may cause extreme fatigue, or loss of strength and stamina.

When thinking about death and funerals, people often think of last rites and paying last respects. While the funeral is clearly a time to recognize a person's life, it is just as much for the family in terms of the grieving and closure process. When we are faced with death, we become more aware of our own mortality and give consideration to our own destiny. Whenever possible, I suggest that a funeral should be a time of celebration.

When death occurs, expect that you will face pain from your loss. Know that you will go through a grieving process that takes time. I love what Max Lucado says about grief: *"As long as your situation brings you no grief, you will receive no comfort."*

People experience grief differently. There is no right or wrong grieving process. So why do we grieve? In the book *Wild at Heart*, John Eldredge states:

> *"It was not your fault and it did matter. Oh what a milestone day that was for me when I simply allowed myself to say that the loss of my father mattered. The tears that flowed were the first I'd ever granted my wound, and they were deeply healing. All those years of sucking it up melted away in my grief. It is so important for us to grieve our wound; it is the only honest thing to do. For in the grieving we admit the truth — that we were hurt by someone we loved, that we lost something very dear, and it hurt us very much. Tears are healing. They help to open and cleanse the wound ... Grief is a form of validation, it says the wound mattered."*

As you experience the grieving process, I encourage you to seek support from within your church, talk with others who have recently lost a loved one and seek resources to help you cope with death. The bookstores are filled with books on the topic of death and dying. You may also choose to talk with a professional counselor.

Did you know that grieving and mourning are different?

- Grieving is an internal feeling and has to do with a natural process individuals go through as they come to accept and work through loss.

- Mourning is the external display of feelings and typically involves events and activities that involve a group of people such as a visitation or funeral.

When the people realized that Aaron had died, all Israel mourned for him thirty days. — **Numbers 20:29 (NLT)**

Faith and Eternal Life

Why, you do not even know what will happen tomorrow. What is your life? You are a mist that appears for a little while and then vanishes. — **James 4:14**

Everything about this life is temporary, even the memory that we ever lived is erased over time.

There is no remembrance of men of old, and even those who are yet to come will not be remembered by those who follow. — **Ecclesiastes 1:11**

The real issue in our lives is the disposition of someone's soul. As loved ones' age or become ill, talk about heaven and salvation. Some people have a false understanding of how we get to heaven. Being a good person is not the correct answer. After all, what is being good? Usually it is comparative — *"I'm better than that person."*

Salvation is based on belief in Jesus Christ. Do you know if your loved one has accepted Jesus into his or her heart? Has your aging family member accepted Jesus Christ as their Lord and Savior? I have heard many people express an uncertainty about their loved one's final destiny.

Do not assume a loved one is saved just because he or she goes to church. Share your faith and what Jesus means to you. Ask about his or her relationship with Christ Jesus. If you are not certain that a loved one is saved, take the opportunity to share the gospel and to reinforce the love of Christ and His promise for those who believe. Encourage the person to accept Jesus Christ as his or her Lord and Savior and offer to lead the person in a prayer of salvation.

Timing matters. Do not wait until tomorrow —tomorrow is not certain. **Do not miss the opportunity**! Do not let a loved one miss out on the eternal life that God offers us.

Likewise, if you are confident about your loved one's salvation, glorify God and give thanks for the promise of eternal life. Find comfort in the fact that you will once again be with your loved ones in heaven.

Reflection and Discussion

Have you spent adequate time preparing for and giving consideration to the death of your parents or loved ones? What are a few things you might consider over the coming weeks and months?

What are the legacies your loved ones will be remembered by once they are gone? What are three or four key points that sum up your life that will be left as your legacy?

Are you aware of your loved ones wishes in terms of the disposition of their body? Are their wishes consistent with yours? Does that present any challenges you would like to share?

What indications are there that your loved one is a believer and is saved? What concerns do you have about the salvation of your loved one? What are some ways you might express your concerns?

List the names of five people you'd like to share the Gospel with over the course of the next few months. Ask God to create a divine appointment when you can share your story of how God touched your life.

KEY LEARNINGS – *Top three findings from this chapter:*
1.
2.
3.

ACTION ITEMS - *Things you want to do or do differently:*

Check when Completed	*Action Item*	*Target Completion Date*

Prayer

Lord God, thank you for Your majesty and sovereignty. Thank you for Your incredible words to guide us along our caregiving journey as we honor the family members and friends we have the privilege of serving. Help us Lord to turn to You for strength and understanding as we face each new challenge. Help us to be a model for our children as we come to realize the very same principles You have shared with us, will some day apply to us, as we are cared for. Grant us peace as we face the realities of aging and death. And most of all Lord, encourage us to share our saving faith and have comfort that our loved ones are being called home to enjoy the splendor that awaits us with You in heaven. In Jesus' name, and for His sake. Amen.

Peace and Purpose

8.
Resources and References

I sincerely hope this book has been a blessing to you!

Please help us to share God's strength, hope and purpose to those who are caregivers and care receivers. I pray that you will suggest this book and share this ministry with your friends and the leadership at your church. In addition, I hope that others within your community will be blessed and find our resources to be of tremendous value.

AGING AMERICA RESOURCES is a 501(c)(3) nonprofit organization devoted to equipping, empowering and encouraging family, pastoral and professional caregivers. We provide action-oriented educational resources that offer practical and spiritual guidance on caring for one another. Our resources, programs, and other supports help caregivers develop the knowledge and skills they need to embrace caregiving and make a difference in the lives of the aging and chronically ill. In addition to offering articles, books, monthly newsletters, small group curriculum and workshops, we provide links to other websites that you might find to be helpful.

People who read CARE For One Another may also find my other two books to be informative and to offer helpful insight:

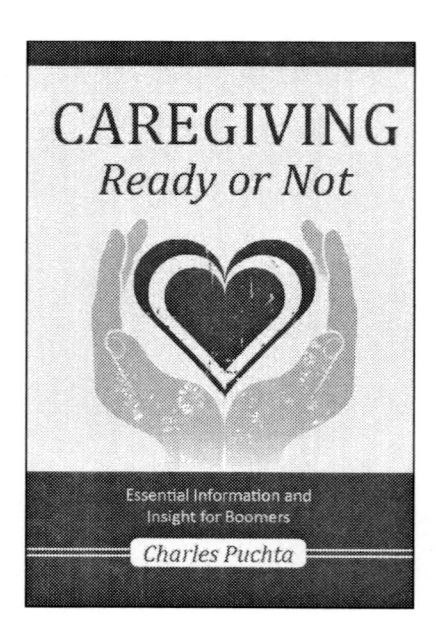

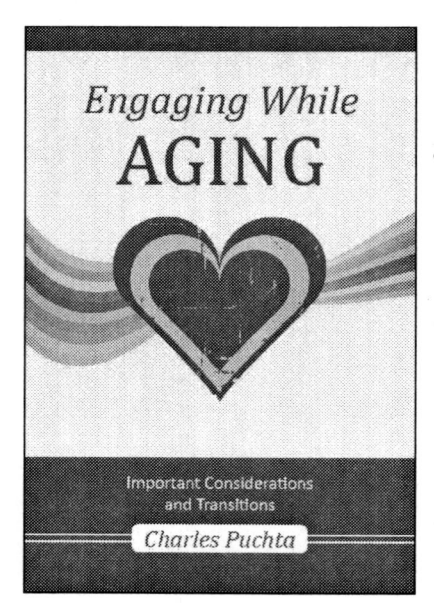

CAREGIVING *Ready or Not* provides the foundational understanding that caregivers so desperately need. The journey I take you through in this book starts with helping you make sense of your situation, discovering your roles and responsibilities, exploring the aging process and seeing life through the lens of a care receiver. Midway through the book I delve deeper into practical and purposeful caregiving, address discussions, decisions and dynamics along with conflict communication strategies. Then I wrap things up addressing loss and grieving, sharing end-of-life considerations, and ideas to help ensure lasting memories. These are all topics caregivers need to know and understand, as doing so will help them engage in more meaningful and supportive ways.

Resources and References

***Engaging While* AGING** addresses important considerations and transitions that older adults need to be prepared for, and baby boomers should begin considering, assuming they have not already done so. I begin this book with a look at the affects of aging, ways to age well and how to minimize safety risks. Knowing that older adults and people with chronic and life-threatening illnesses are likely to encounter many important and difficult decisions, I address the issues they are likely to face, explain the common concerns, explain the various options that might be available and offer advice to help people avoid surprises. In this book I cover topics such as driving/transportation, and living environments and care arrangement. I offer insight and share information everyone needs to know about advance directives, legal and financial planning. I address government services, insurance options, Hospice care, funeral planning, the handling of personal belongings, and more. *(Available February '10.)*

For more information about Aging America Resources, to order books, inquire about speaking engagements, or to make a donation to this ministry, our contact information is:

>Aging America Resources
>11611 Kosine Lane, Suite 101
>Loveland, OH 45140
>
>Website: www.Caregiving.CC
>
>Phone: (513) 377-7965

Other Suggested Resources

LIVING FREE / Turning Point Ministries offers small group resources, daily devotionals and more. All of their resources help people turn to God when dealing with life's problems.

Caregiving: Caring for Aging Parents is a small group curriculum written by Charles Puchta and published by Living Free/ Turning Point Ministries. The study addresses the predominate issues most families face as loved ones age or become ill. Each lesson is divided into Self-Awareness and Spiritual-Awareness sections. Both a Facilitator's Guide and Group Member's Guide are available. To learn more or to purchase *Caregiving: Caring for Aging Parents* or other small group curriculums offered by Living Free/Turning Point Ministries, visit www.LivingFree.CC or call (800) 879-4770.

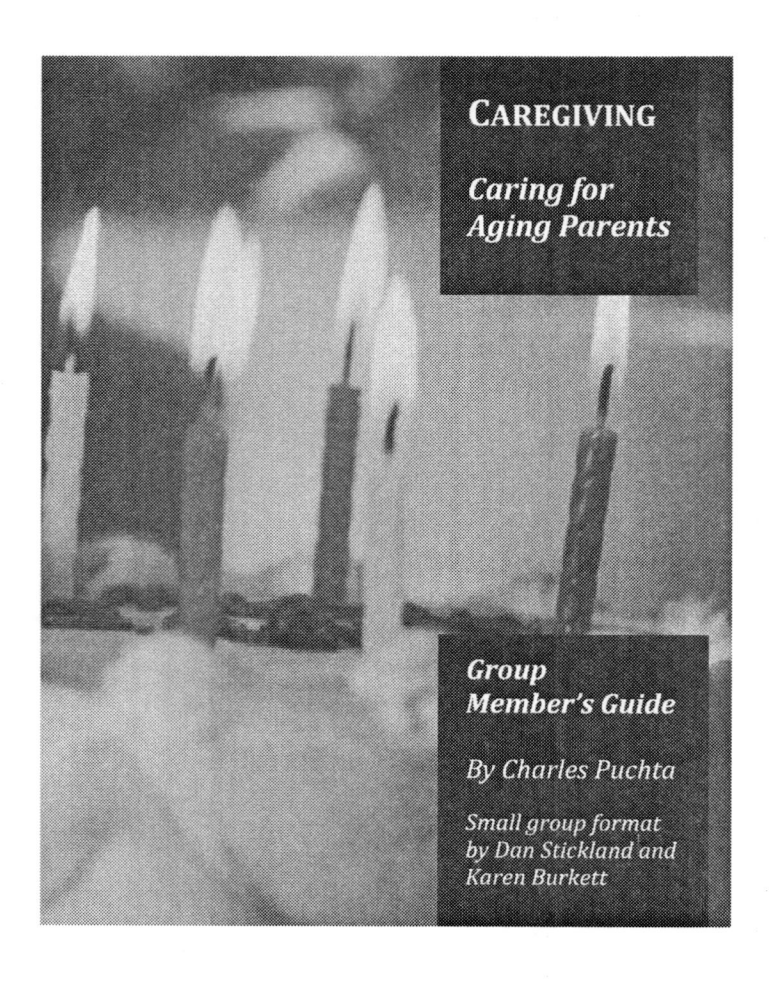

CENTER FOR AGING WITH DIGNITY – The Center for Aging with Dignity at the University of Cincinnati College of Nursing is devoted to keeping people *SAFE After 60* by advocating for, advancing and developing best-practice programs on the safety and mistreatment of older adults. Recognizing that safety risks increase with age, we focus on enhancing the ability of professionals to empower older adults, families and organizations to maximize heath, wellness and independence. Charles Puchta, author of this book is the Center director. For more information visit www.SafeAfter60.CC

References

Administration in Aging, U.S. Department of Health and Human Services. (2008). *Profile of Older Adults: 2008* retrieved from http://www.aoa.gov/AoAroot/Aging_Statistics/Profile/2008/docs/2008profile.pdf.

Arterburn. S. & Stoop, D. (1991) *The Angry Man*. Nashville: W Publishing Group

Bee, H. L. (2000) *The Journey of Adulthood* (4th ed., pp. 62-97). Upper Saddle River, NJ: Prentice Hall.

Chapman, G. (2004). *The Five Love Languages*. Chicago: Northfield Publishing.

Duka, W. (2004, March). Will Your Ship Come In? AARP Bulletin. Retrieved from http://www.aarp.org/bulletin/yourmoney/Articles/a2004-02-26-ship.html

Eldredge, J. (2006) *Wild at Heart*. Nashville: Thomas Nelson.

Hybels, B. (1987). Who Are You When No One's Looking. Downers Grove, IL: InterVarsity Press.

National Institute on Aging. (2002, January). *Age Page: Taking Care of Your Teeth and Mouth* retrieved from http://www.niapublications.org/agepages/teeth.asp

Phelan, E. A., & Larson, E. B. (2002). "Successful Aging" – Where Next? *Journal of the American Geriatrics Society, 50*:1306-1308.

Puchta, C. (2007). *Caregiving, Caring for Aging Parents*. Chattanooga, TN: Living Free/Turning Point Ministries.